CNOR® Exam Study Guide

2nd Edition

*Produced by CCI, the
official governing body of the
CNOR® certification program*

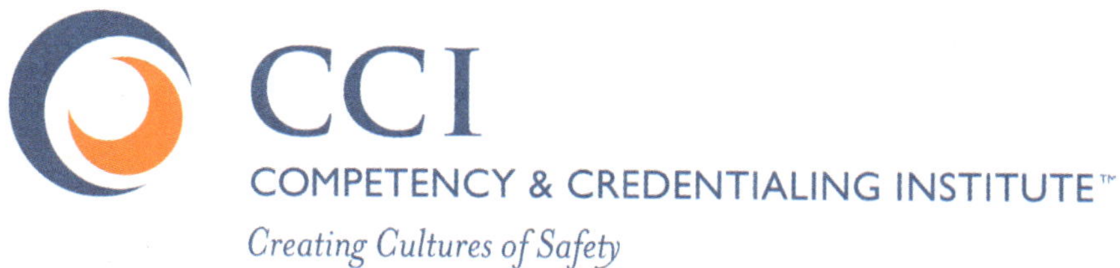

Published by
Competency & Credentialing Institute
2170 South Parker Road, Suite 295
Denver, CO 80231

CNOR® Exam Study Guide

2nd Edition

Produced by CCI, the official governing body of the CNOR certification program

This preparation guide has been developed to provide resources and guidance for the perioperative nurse who is preparing for the CNOR examination. The perioperative nurse's scope of practice has been used as the overall basis for the organization of this publication and also serves as the basic framework for each chapter.

The Competency & Credentialing Institute presents this publication to enhance the knowledge and skill level of the perioperative nurse who strives to demonstrate achievement in practice. Using this book as a study guide, however, is not required, nor does it guarantee successfully passing the exam.

Table of Contents

PREFACE

Julie Mower, MSN, RN, CNS, CNOR
Credentialing and Education Project Manager
Competency & Credentialing Institute

Earning the CNOR® credential is a highly sought after professional and personal goal. As a certified perioperative nurse, you demonstrate your competency every day in support of quality patient care. CCI wants to help you achieve this professional milestone by providing materials to help you prepare for your certification exam.

The *CNOR Exam Study Guide* is just one of many tools that CCI offers as an aid to your preparation for the CNOR examination. Depending on your level of experience, it may be necessary to access other resources in addition to this book, because the CNOR exam is a comprehensive assessment of every facet of perioperative nursing practice.

This *Guide* is designed to build on your current knowledge and experience by providing opportunities to engage in critical-thinking exercises. Interactive learning activities ask you to apply current best practices to common clinical situations encountered by a nurse with two years of experience. It is highly recommended that you use the references cited in each module to complete the exercises in this book. The answers to the questions on the CNOR exam are based on these same references.

Before you start reviewing the material, please note that this *Guide* contains features that help to make it a more useful preparation tool. These include:

- A section titled "How To Use This Book" that outlines the book format and learning activities (page 11).

- A section titled "Strategies for Success: Getting Prepared and Being Test-Wise" to help you prepare to take the exam. You will find information on the process involved in answering multiple-choice questions and test-taking strategies from an exam development expert (page 16).

- A self-assessment to help you evaluate your current knowledge and skills and guide you in developing your own study plan (page 28).

- A learning needs assessment that matches current knowledge with content on the exam (page 31).

- A study plan with a suggested template for organizing and focusing on key components of the exam (Appendix A, pages 267-272).

- A CD that contains master forms used in the learning activities so that additional copies may be made; 50 of the popular "Questions of the Week" with detailed answers and additional references, taken from CCI's Perioperative Question of the Week on Facebook (http://www.facebook.com/PeriopQuestion?v=app_4949752878); and instructions for completing a concept map.

- A list of the domains covered in the exam, with pertinent topics listed under each domain to help guide your studying (Appendix B, pages 273-282).

Studies show that people retain more information when they use an interactive learning approach that includes reading the information, talking about it, and writing it. We encourage you to use this workbook as the basis for studying with a group of your peers and fellow exam-takers. You may also want to contact a CCI Champion in your institution for guidance. CCI Champions understand the value of certification and help mentor nurses seeking the CNOR credential. A list of Champions is available on our web site (www.cc-institute.org) under the "Champions" tab.

If you have questions about this *Guide* or preparing for the CNOR exam, please contact CCI at (888) 257-2667. ***Good luck as you embark on this exciting phase of your career.***

Contributing Authors

Julie Mower, MSN, RN, CNS, CNOR
Project Manager
Competency & Credentialing Institute
Denver, Colorado

Terri Goodman, PhD, RN, CNOR
Consultant
Terri Goodman and Associates
Dallas, Texas

Jane Fulton-Junge, BSN, RN
Perioperative Educator
St. Anthony Central Hospital
Denver, Colorado

Linda D. Waters, PhD, RN
Vice President
Prometric
Baltimore, Maryland

Reviewers

Chris Kennedy, BSN, MA, RN, CNOR
Nurse Informaticist
Lawrence and Memorial Hospital
New London, Connecticut

Constance Melby, MS, RN, CNOR
Manager, Bettendorf Surgical Services
Trinity Medical Center
Bettendorf, Iowa

Kathi Knipfer, MS, RN, CNOR
Clinical Educator, Perioperative Services
Exempla Good Samaritan Medical Center
Lafayette, Colorado

Kathryn Schroeter, PhD, RN, CNOR
Assistant Professor, College of Nursing
Marquette University
Milwaukee, Wisconsin

Lisa Spruce, DNP, RN, ACNP-BC, ANP-BC, ACNS-BC, CNOR
Corporate Clinical Manager of Surgery
Universal Health Services
King of Prussia, Pennsylvania

Jan Stull, MS, RN, CNOR
Perioperative Educator
Porter Adventist Hospital
Denver, Colorado

Julia Thompson, PhD, RN, APRN, CIP, CNOR
Administrative Director, Research and Sponsored Programs
Harris County Hospital District
Houston, Texas

Susan Younger, MNA, RN, CNOR
Service Leader, Procedure Center
The Children's Hospital
Aurora, Colorado

Graphics
Larin Zamora
Littleton, Colorado

Note: Concept maps created with templates from https://bubbl.us.

INTRODUCTION

Overview

This book is probably different from other study guides you may have used to prepare for exams. It certainly is different from previous *Guides to CNOR Exam Preparation.* Instead of providing a summary of a specific topic with sample test questions, the format has been reversed — you are expected to bring the knowledge accrued from your years of experience and your readings of recommended reference materials, and apply it to problem-based scenarios and questions that are based on actual clinical situations. These learning activities should not be considered all-inclusive for what will be covered on the exam; rather, they should be viewed as "brain templates," or a way to approach problem-solving any clinical issue. It is hoped that this active thinking process will serve you well, not only for the purposes of studying for the exam, but also in your professional practice. After all, passing the exam is just the beginning, not the end, of your continued quest for competence.

Getting Ready: References and Resources

Hypothetically, if one has experience with a variety of types of cases in a work environment that supports current best practices, it may not be necessary to study for the exam at all. Your practice would already mirror the correct answers on the exam. However, most of us feel more secure reviewing the topics that will be covered on the exam. It's important to remember that the exam is based on best practices as reflected in the current literature, which may differ from the clinical practice at any one facility.

Although there are many quality perioperative resources available on the market today, both this *Guide* and the exam are based on information found in four key reference books. Use the most current edition of each of these books for studying. Best practices change over time (how many of us remember doing a pre-op shave for our patient the night before surgery?), and you will not save money by purchasing or borrowing outdated materials and possibly jeopardizing your chances of successfully passing the exam.

Reading assignments from these books are included at the beginning of each module in this guide. Using these books will help you respond to the learning activities and prepare for the content covered on the exam.

Required Reference

- AORN. (2013). *Perioperative Standards and Recommended Practices*. Denver.

This is the primary resource that guides our perioperative practice. It may be purchased at www.aorn.org. Being a member of AORN allows you to purchase this book, as well as other references in their bookstore, at a discount. Members also receive a discount on the CNOR exam application fee. Supporting AORN is an important part of our responsibility as professional perioperative nurses. Along with the CNOR credential, it demonstrates a commitment to quality, safe patient care.

Highly Recommended References

Any of the following will be sufficient; it is not necessary to purchase all of them.

- Rothrock, J. (ed.). (2011). *Alexander's Care of the Patient in Surgery*. St. Louis: Mosby Elsevier.

- Phillips, N. (ed.). (2013). *Berry and Kohn's Operating Room Technique*. St. Louis: Mosby Elsevier.

- Phippen, M., Ulmer, B., & Wells, M. (2009). *Competency for Safe Patient Care During Operative and Invasive Procedures*. Denver: CCI.

Depending on your clinical practice, you may want to supplement these books with additional resources on pharmacology, pathophysiology, or diagnostic/lab values. Space prevents a more extensive list, but a sampling of recently published books is provided below. This list is not all-inclusive, and there are many other good references available. It's important to find a book that is easy for you to use and that contains the most current information available.

Pathophysiology

- McCance, K.L., Huether, S.E. (2010). *Pathophysiology: The Biologic Basis for Disease in Adults and Children*. Maryland Heights, MO: Mosby Elsevier.

> **Tip for Success**
>
> Before going through the expense of purchasing any of these books, see if you can borrow references from your facility library, unit manager, perioperative educator, or other staff members who may either have recently taken the exam or are in the process of studying.

- Porth, C. (2011). *Essentials of Pathophysiology: Concepts of Altered Health States*. Philadelphia, PA: Wolters Kluwer Health/Lippincott Williams and Wilkin.

Laboratory/Diagnostic Tests

- Kee, J. L. (2013). *Laboratory and Diagnostic Tests with Nursing Implications*. Upper Saddle River, NJ: Prentice Hall.

- Pagana, K.D. & Pagana, T.J. (2013). *Mosby's Manual of Diagnostic and Laboratory Tests*. St. Louis: Mosby Elsevier.

Pharmacology

- Vallerand, A., & Sanoski, C. (2013). *Davis' Drug Guide for Nurses*. Philadelphia, PA: F.A. Davis.

- Lacy, C.F., Armstrong, L.L., Goldman, M.P., & Lance, L.L. (eds.). *Drug Information Handbook 2013-2014: A Comprehensive Resource for All Clinicians and Healthcare Professionals*. Philadelphia: Lexicomp, Inc./Wolters Kluwer Health.

> **Tip for Success**
>
> Your facility may already have an online formulary available for you to use at no cost. An excellent online resource is epocrates (https://online.epocrates.com/home). It's free, is updated frequently, and can be downloaded to your PDA or smart phone.

Nursing Diagnoses

- AORN. (2011). *Perioperative Nursing Data Set*. Denver.

Making This Guide Work for You

Each chapter in this guide is based on a domain, or topic, found on the exam. The format of this book encourages you to write in it, reflect on your progress, and identify your strengths and areas for improvement. Make it your own. Each chapter is organized as follows.

The *percentage of questions* on a particular domain is found at the beginning of the chapter. If study time is in short supply, this may help you organize your time by focusing on the chapters with the highest percentage of questions.

Modules are organized based on the tasks and knowledge statements found in each domain (see Appendix B). They help organize the "chunks" of information and make the process of studying more manageable.

Competency outcomes are provided for successfully completing the chapter. This allows you to quickly check to see if you already know the content, or will need to review it.

Detailed *reading assignments* cover the content for the domain. This information will also be used to complete the learning activities.

Key words help to further focus your reading on relevant content.

Case study activities are based on our sample patient, introduced in Chapter 1.

Learning activities require application of the content from the reading assignments and prerequisite knowledge and skills. These learning activities may be any combination of short answer, fill in the blank, multiple choice, or scenario-based.

Skill building activities encourage you to take advantage of additional learning opportunities in your clinical setting.

The *summary* at the end of each chapter provides "golden rules" for competent practice.

A *glossary* at the end of each chapter defines words or terms that may be unfamiliar. Answers to learning activities are provided at the end of each chapter.

Additional *readings and resources* are included at the end of each module.

How to Use the CD

The CD contains supplemental information to enhance the activities in the workbook. Instructions on how to develop a concept map (introduced in Chapter 1), perioperative questions that encourage dialogue with your peers and critical thinking, and blank templates for many of the forms found in your book are additional learning tools.

A Note on Taking Practice Tests

Many people like to use sample tests as part of their studying routine. This is in no way a requirement for successfully passing the exam. If you decide to purchase practice questions, the following information will be helpful in maximizing their usefulness.

The purposes of the sample test questions are twofold: to provide an experience similar to taking the actual CNOR exam, and to evaluate your knowledge of a particular topic. These multiple-choice questions are comparable in form and content to the types of questions on the actual CNOR certification exam. If testing anxiety is a concern, completing the practice test should mirror the actual exam as closely as possible. Resist the urge to immediately look up the answer to each question. You won't be able to do this on the actual exam, which may be a source of additional anxiety on testing day.

Many nurses find answering practice test questions helpful in preparing for the exam, but it is important to understand this tool's limitations. First, these questions WILL NOT be found on the actual exam. The practice questions should not be used as a substitute for studying. Answering the sample questions multiple times has limited benefit, as you will begin to memorize not only the answers, but the questions, which diminishes their value as a tool to evaluate what you know or don't know. Other tips for utilizing the practice questions to their fullest potential:

- For all the questions, look up the rationale in your text books, whether you answered the question correctly or not. Active involvement in the learning process means you'll be more likely to remember the content, and provides the "why" that you can then apply to similar questions.

- Look at trends; missing multiple questions in a single domain (for example, preoperative assessment or emergency situations) means extra studying and/or clinical exposure is needed in those areas.

- Take the "big picture" view of incorrect answers; missing a question on a particular drug means you will want to review that drug, but it may also signify a knowledge deficit in pharmacology in general.

It is important to remember that the level of success in answering the practice questions in no way transfers to success on the actual exam. More preparation ideas for test-taking can be found in CCI's *CNOR Candidate Handbook* (www.cc-institute.org) and in the next section.

Guide to Activities

Several types of activities are included in this *Guide*. Activities to be completed within the printed book include matching, fill-in-the blank, and other types of exercises. An example of a matching activity is shown at the right.

Activities that require the learner to seek outside information or perform tasks outside the printed book (e.g., on the CD) are called "Go To" Activities and appear in a framed box.

Exercises related to the Case Study introduced in Chapter One are labeled as such and outlined in orange.

Activity — Matching
EXAMPLE: From the list of patient assessment data below, write . . .

"Go To" Activity
EXAMPLE: On the CD, go to Question #6, . . .

Case Study Activity
EXAMPLE: How does Mrs. M.'s allergy to penicillin affect . . .

Let's Get Started!

By now you are either excited about starting on your journey to validate your practice as a competent perioperative nurse, or are overwhelmed at the magnitude of the task ahead. Both emotions are totally normal. Just remember that the test is based on what a nurse with two years of practice is expected to know. As a person eligible to take the exam, you already have met this criterion. So... let's get started!

Strategies for Success: Getting Prepared and Being Test-Wise

Contributing author: Linda D. Waters, PhD, RN

Being successful at passing the CNOR certification examination for perioperative nursing requires having a thorough and sound foundation of the knowledge and skills required for competent clinical practice, as well as an understanding of the test-taking process. Knowledge is attained through work experiences and independent learning, as well as through formal educational programs. The experiential knowledge component requires that an individual who is eligible to take the CNOR certification examination has a minimum of two years of work experience in perioperative nursing. The knowledge component is acquired through a variety of learning activities, including formal education, self-study, and continuing education programs, all aiming to promote continuing competency. It is the combination of experiential and cognitive knowledge that forms the foundation of competent clinical practice.

In addition to evidence-based clinical knowledge, you will also need to have a firm understanding of the testing process. Being familiar with the testing process will not only prepare you to take the test and enable you to feel more confident about the testing experience, but will also acquaint you with the environment in which the test will be given. There is a definite skill in answering multiple-choice test questions. Becoming familiar with techniques for responding to multiple-choice questions will improve your chances of successful performance on the CNOR certification examination.

This chapter provides information about planning your personalized study program, obtaining the necessary resources to assist in your preparation, understanding the processes involved with answering multiple-choice test questions, and developing sound test-taking strategies to lead to success on your CNOR certification examination.

Learning Objectives

Upon completion of this section, the individual will be able to:

1. Identify specific content areas in perioperative nursing where further study is needed.
2. Develop an action plan and timeline for acquiring additional knowledge in content areas where needed.
3. Identify resources that will be of assistance in preparing for the CNOR certification examination.
4. Identify the major features of multiple-choice test questions.
5. Develop skill in applying test-taking strategies when answering multiple-choice test questions.
6. Plan a success-oriented action plan for taking the CNOR certification examination.

Developing Good Study Habits

Making the initial commitment to take a certification examination is an important decision. For most test takers, becoming certified in a specialty area of nursing practice accomplishes both personal and professional goals. The personal goal is a feeling of accomplishment — tackling a task that may be difficult yet, at the same time, rewarding. Professionally, certification provides external recognition of excellence in nursing and may promote career advancement. In addition, certification is a symbol of achievement that distinguishes the credential holder from others in the field. The certification holder can proudly state that he or she has met a high standard of achievement established by experts in nursing. It is truly an accomplishment to acquire certification as a CNOR.

The next step in the certification process is determining what your personal investment will be in preparing for the examination. And what a personal investment it is! Perhaps the easiest actions are completing the application and paying the examination fee. The more difficult part is realistically determining what you want to do and can do to prepare for the examination. Each person will need to decide what works best for him or her. Ultimately, when you go to take your examination, you want to be certain you are as prepared as you can be and are confident about your ability to demonstrate your command of perioperative nursing knowledge.

Preparing to take the CNOR examination may seem like an overwhelming task. Answering the following questions may help organize your study plan.

Question #1 — Should I study for the examination?

Studying for the examination is your choice and is, in no small way, a decision based on your years of experience in perioperative nursing. While experience is critical, your personal work experiences may not have provided you with the broad range of skills and knowledge needed to be successful on the certification examination. Remember, a certification examination is a general examination that will ask questions about many areas of perioperative nursing. Ask yourself whether your experiences in perioperative nursing have been broad enough to prepare you for all content areas that might be included on the test. Are there areas of practice with which you have not had work experience or where standards of practice may have recently changed?

So, do you need to study? Conduct a self-assessment to determine your chances for passing the certification examination. How do you do that?

An excellent starting point is to review critical documents, including the *CNOR Candidate Handbook*, found at www.cc-institute.org; the CNOR Exam Study Plan; and the current AORN *Perioperative Standards and Recommended Practices*. Turn to page 31 to complete your learning needs assessment. Assess your "level of competency" for each content area. Conduct this assessment before you register and schedule your examination to allow sufficient preparation time before the examination. Use a rating scale such as the one below to determine what you believe to be your current level of competency.

1 — Very Certain: I know this content area well and believe that my work experiences have fully prepared me. I am comfortable with current practices and believe I am up-to-date with new developments and advances.

2 — Certain: I am reasonably comfortable with this content area and believe that my work experiences have prepared me fairly well.

3 — Undecided: I have some knowledge and some experiences in this area, but there may be a few content areas where I am not as strong or for which my work experiences have not fully prepared me. I may not be current in all areas of perioperative nursing.

4 — Uncertain: I am aware that I have some knowledge deficits and/or a lack of work experience in this content area. I will need to engage in some study or other remediation to be comfortable with this content area.

5 — Very Uncertain: I am aware that I have many knowledge deficits and/or lack work experiences in this content area. These areas of weakness will require me to engage in remediation activities before taking the examination.

Apply this rating scale to each domain of the *CNOR Candidate Handbook*. Be completely honest with your learning assessment — remember, it is intended to help you prepare for the CNOR examination. If you rate all areas as 1 or 2, you may find that you will need little to no preparation before taking the examination. If, on the other hand, you find that you have a mixture of responses, rating some 1 and 2 and others 3, 4, or 5, you may find it very useful to develop an individualized study plan that will allow you sufficient time to prepare before taking the examination. Appendix B (pages 273-282) has a more detailed breakdown of subjects included in each section, or domain, of the exam.

Knowing that you have done all you can to prepare for taking the CNOR certification examination will give you that extra boost of confidence! It also will help you determine when to schedule your examination within the testing period.

Be realistic! Preparing for the examination will be best completed over a period of weeks, not days or hours. Unexpected events will occur which may take away from your preparation time. Don't shortchange yourself. Allow sufficient study time before the examination.

Question #2 — What is the most important content to study?

Go back to the learning needs assessment you completed when making the decision whether to study. Consider dividing the content areas from the *CNOR Candidate Handbook* into three broad areas:

Area 1 — Content that I have knowledge strengths.

Area 2 — Content that is mixed; I may know some areas but have weaknesses in others.

Area 3 — Content that I know I have knowledge weaknesses.

Then look at the proportion of the test that is dedicated to each area you identified (Appendix C, page 283). Concentrate your study time on those areas where you have the greatest knowledge weaknesses and where the largest percentage of test questions will be represented. Tackle those needs FIRST, before going on to other areas. Each chapter in this interactive guide outlines the percentage of questions found on that topic on the examination.

Question #3 — What is the best study style for me?

Once you have decided that you do want to study for the examination and you have developed a study plan specific to your needs, next determine a study style that works best for you. Remember back to your school days. What worked best for you then? Were you more successful when you studied alone in the privacy of your own study space? Or were you more focused when you studied with others? Maybe a combination study style works best for you — individual study for reviewing familiar concepts and group study for learning new content areas.

What will likely be different now from your earlier study experiences in high school or college is the amount of time you have available for study. Looking back, those earlier days were a lot easier when you had fewer commitments. As you prepare for your certification examination you must balance your other commitments (e.g., family, work) with your need to prepare for the examination.

Plan the best time for taking the examination. If you know that the next few months are especially busy for you with unusual work expectations (e.g., staff shortages, preparing for an accreditation visit) or family responsibilities (e.g., vacation, childcare, holidays), don't add to these burdens by scheduling the examination during that period. Remember, you have the flexibility to choose a testing time that works best for you.

Because the CNOR certification examination is available Monday through Saturday throughout the year, register and schedule the examination at a time that is best for you — a time that allows you adequate preparation and no other major commitments or conflicts. Please visit the CCI website (www.cc-institute.org) for current testing deadlines and windows.

Remember, this certification examination is important for you both personally and professionally. Once you have made the commitment to take the examination, commit also to developing a personalized study plan — and stick to it! Engage help from your family, friends, and colleagues to stick to your study plan.

Question #4 — How do I plan and manage my study time?

Once you have completed your learning needs assessment and identified what you need to study, you will be able to develop a study schedule that, if adhered to, should guide you to a successful testing experience. Study to your weaknesses. Obviously, the more knowledge weaknesses you identify in major areas that will be covered on the CNOR certification examination, the greater time you will need to allow for fulfilling your study schedule.

Most important is to stay focused and committed to your study plan. You will be most confident if you plan for your study time and stick to the study schedule you develop. Use your study time wisely. Make use of any spare time that you have to review concepts.

Here are some suggestions to make the best use of your study time.

- Make a timeline, based on the date for your examination, which outlines specific daily and weekly study time commitments. Make sure your timeline takes into account personal lifestyle issues (work schedule, holidays, family responsibilities, etc.) that will impact the time available to study.

- Set a study schedule and stick with it. Use the study plan found in Appendix A (pages 267-272) to help you organize your time. Engage the help of friends and family to help you stay focused and motivated.

- Prepare a work area where you can leave your study materials so that they are readily available.

- Try to study a little every day, instead of long sessions sporadically; you'll retain more, and it gives you more opportunities to review the material. Repetition is important for learning.

Question #5 — What do I study?

A list of recommended references is found in the study plan and in the introduction to this book. Don't forget online resources that provide additional sources of study materials. There are excellent resources that can be found through the Internet. Consider combining your study preparation with earning continuing education credit. Complete continuing education programs that can be found online, or simply call up a topic of interest and search the Internet to see what is available.

Handy Study Tips

- Consider making flashcards out of index cards and carry those with you everywhere. You can turn even an extra five minutes into valuable study time.

- Balance "old" learning with "new" learning. As you prepare for the examination, you will find some content areas where you need to simply review or "brush up" on your knowledge. In other cases, you may discover "new" content areas that you will need to learn. Remember that the examination is a general examination of perioperative nursing, and the content areas evaluated by the examination may include areas in which you have not previously worked. Try to balance your study sessions to allow some new knowledge gains along with the review of more familiar content.

- Use your work setting as your personal learning lab. In some ways, each workday provides you with an excellent opportunity to prepare for the examination. See how you can build in new knowledge in your daily activities. For example, are you administering a drug that is not used frequently? Use that opportunity to go to a reference and learn more about the drug. Are you assisting in a new surgical procedure? Ask questions of your colleagues and find out all you can, especially about areas that are less familiar to you.

- Let your work colleagues know that you are preparing for your certification examination. Sharing your plans to take the certification examination with your work colleagues will accomplish two purposes. First, ask them to "remind" you that you need to prepare for the examination. Your colleagues can be a great source of support and encouragement. Give them the "okay" to ask you if you are on schedule with your preparation. Second, ask your colleagues to become your study coaches. Remind them to seek you out when they have an interesting surgical case or when there is a new learning opportunity. You may want to share with your colleagues the areas where you believe you have knowledge weaknesses so they can be on the alert for study opportunities that relate.

Stay focused on your goal. At some point in your study cycle, you will no doubt ask yourself, "Why did I decide to do this?" It is normal to feel a bit overwhelmed, but sticking to your goal will be rewarding.

Components of a Multiple-Choice Test Question

In addition to a planned study program, you should work to develop your knowledge and skill in answering multiple-choice questions. It is important that you understand the structure and format of this type of test question.

The CNOR certification examination is comprised of multiple-choice questions, written by experts in perioperative nursing. As such, each question is written to assess important knowledge and skills essential for competent perioperative nursing practice. Much effort goes into developing each question, including multiple reviews by many subject matter experts. Questions are never designed to "trick" the test taker. Rather, questions are designed to differentiate test takers who know the content from those who do not.

Each question on the examination is a four-option, multiple-choice test question (or item). A multiple-choice test question consists of the stem and the options. The stem provides the information that supports the question that is being asked. It should contain sufficient information for you to understand what is being asked, even by just reading it alone.

The stem is followed by four options, one of which is the correct answer (or key) as determined by a panel of content experts and validated by current literature. The other three options are the distracters, which are plausible but not correct answers. There is one and only one correct answer among the options provided.

The stem of each test question may be closed-ended or open-ended. A closed-ended question asks a complete question and ends with a question mark. An open-ended question is a type of fill-in-the-blank with the four choices provided as the options. Each of the choices will complete the statement.

The following are examples of each question format:

Closed-ended question:

Which of the following is the rationale for having perioperative nursing personnel immunized with hepatitis B vaccine?
1. Current legislation requires the immunization.
2. Occupational risk of acquiring the hepatitis virus is high. (Correct answer)
3. The immunization also provides protection against other forms of hepatitis.
4. Standard precautions require routine immunization for all bloodborne viruses.

Open-ended question:

Perioperative nursing personnel should receive hepatitis B immunization because:
1. current legislation requires the immunization.
2. the occupational risk of acquiring the hepatitis virus is high. (Correct answer)
3. the immunization also provides protection against other forms of hepatitis.
4. standard precautions require routine immunization for all bloodborne viruses.

The multiple-choice test questions used in the CNOR certification examination measure either basic knowledge or pose a situation where an application of the knowledge is required. Because clinical practice requires the ability to apply principles and facts to patient situations, most of the test questions on the CNOR certification examination are at the application level. The following are examples of these two types of questions:

Knowledge/Comprehension:

The loss of heat from exposed body parts due to exposure of air currents is known as:
1. evaporation.

2. conduction.
3. radiation.
4. convection. (Correct answer)

Application:

During skin preparation, the scrub person informs the perioperative nurse that the sleeve of a student's warm-up jacket has brushed against the area being prepared. Which of the following would be an appropriate response for the perioperative nurse to take first?
1. Report the incident to the instructor for follow-up.
2. Have the student review the required technique.
3. Review skin preparation at the next in-service program.
4. Inform the student immediately of the break in technique. (Correct answer)

Before any question is added to the CNOR certification examination, it is "pretested" on a representative group of test takers to ensure that the question is clearly stated, that there is only one correct answer, and that the question performs statistically across all candidates as intended. This occurs before the question is included and scored in an actual test administration.

One point is given for each correct answer. The total score on the examination is the total points given for all correct answers. There is no penalty for guessing, so answer all questions. Budget your time wisely to complete the entire test.

Taking the CNOR Certification Examination

The CNOR certification examination is a computer-based test that is administered at a test center. Each testing candidate schedules an individualized testing appointment for a date and time that is convenient for them. Unlike paper-and-pencil tests where there may be several hundred individuals in the same room, the computer test center is designed to accommodate multiple tests and each person in the testing room may be taking a different examination. Some of these examinations may be shorter or longer than the CNOR certification examination, so you will notice that others either are leaving the room ahead of you or are still taking their examination when you have finished.

When the examination begins, you will first be given a brief on-screen tutorial that will orient you to taking a test on a computer. Remember that you do not need computer skills or familiarity with a computer to take the CNOR certification examination. And, even if you are very skilled in using a computer, the tutorial that is part of the examination will teach you how to navigate within this examination.

While the mouse is more commonly used, the keyboard is enabled for use in answering questions. In addition, the tutorial will provide instructions on using the various features: "Previous," which allows you to return to a previously seen question; "Mark," which allows you to identify specific test questions that you would like to return to at a later time whether you have answered the question or skipped it; and "Review," which presents a list of all of the test questions and highlights those questions that you have marked. As you proceed through the test, you may skip a question and return to it later to answer. You may review questions at any time, or wait until the end of the test.

You should complete the tutorial in its entirety, focusing on how the features of the test operate so that you are familiar with these functions. Your answers to the practice questions in the tutorial are not included in your test score.

The test center staff that proctors the examination and monitors your activities will be located in a viewing area outside the testing room and are available if you need assistance. They are not content experts about perioperative nursing, so they are not able to provide you with any assistance about the test questions themselves. Their role is to monitor the activities in the testing room and report any unusual situations or inappropriate behavior. If you have a concern about a test question, you will have an opportunity to report your concern at the end of the examination.

You will find more information about the testing situation in the *CNOR Candidate Handbook*. In addition, your Authorization to Test (ATT) that will be e-mailed to you includes instructions about the day of the examination, what time to arrive at the testing center, what identification you will need, and other general guidelines.

Hints for Taking Tests

For many individuals, the CNOR certification examination will be the first test taken in many years. The mere thought of sitting for nearly four hours answering multiple-choice questions brings back memories of earlier testing situations. So it is important that you prepare yourself to be in the best physical and mental condition that is possible.

If you have not taken a computer-based test before, search out opportunities to practice using this method. Many hospitals' annual competencies are computer-based. Many continuing education evaluations are also computer-based.

Keep yourself in good physical health before the examination date. You should plan to eat a balanced meal the evening before and then get a good night's sleep. Sleep rather than cram the night before; your critical thinking skills are not based solely on the information you've memorized. Plan to eat breakfast before a morning appointment (or lunch before an afternoon appointment), because you will be in the testing room for 3 hours and 45 minutes. Avoid over-eating though, as too much food or liquids could make you tired. Feeling well and being rested are important strategies for success. You need to be able to read carefully and think clearly.

Some people become anxious about the testing situation and have difficulty focusing and processing complex information. One way to reduce this anxiety is for you to identify those portions of the exam day that are completely in your control. Be sure you know the directions to the testing center and leave ample time for traffic delays. Make certain that the required admissions materials are collected the evening before (see "Day of Test Checklist") and are readily available to you as you leave for your appointment.

Test-Taking Guidelines

Success in passing the certification examination takes more than just knowing the content. You need to understand how to read and answer multiple-choice test questions. There is a very simple and easy-to-follow strategy in taking multiple-choice tests.

When reading multiple-choice test questions, it is important to remember that there is one and only one correct answer. So, consider the following.

- Attempt to answer the question before reading the options, and then look for an option that best fits your answer. You should be able to answer a multiple-choice question without reading the options.

- Cover up the options and see if you can determine an answer to the question being asked. Then, uncover the options. Often you will find that your answer is one of the options provided. In that case, your best course of action is to go with your first answer. Try to avoid changing an answer.

- Note that the options are written to be plausible to those who do not know the content. Well-written multiple-choice questions are designed to have four plausible options. The intent is to discriminate between those candidates who know the information and those who do not. If you are unsure of the answer, try to eliminate options that you believe are incorrect. This improves your chance of selecting the correct answer.

- Eliminate options that have absolutes, such as "always" or "never." There is very little in nursing practice that is absolute. Most courses of action in clinical practice and most client responses are "usually" or "generally."

- Read the question carefully, paying special attention to phrases such as "most," "most appropriate," "primarily," "first," and "initially." Often, all of the options are applicable to the situation, but only one option fits the emphasis included in the stem.

- Answer all of the questions. Credit is given for all correct answers. So if you are unsure of an answer, take an educated guess among the plausible options.

- Monitor your progress by noting the time remaining on the computer screen. The CNOR certification examination is timed to provide you with about one minute per question. If you find that you are taking more time than expected to answer a question, mark the question and return to it once you have finished reading through the entire test. You do not want to spend too much time reading one test question and then run out of time, leaving several questions at the end unanswered. Unanswered questions will be scored as incorrect.

- Review your work after you have completed the test. Once you have read through the test and answered as many questions as you can, you should return to review the questions that you may have skipped or marked for further review. Then, if there is available time when you have completed the entire test, you can review all of the questions and reconsider your choices. You should refrain from making too many changes. Often, test takers change a right response to a wrong response.

How to Avoid Making Errors

Being successful in passing the certification examination requires that you also avoid making mistakes in answering the test questions. One helpful strategy to avoid test-taking errors is to take practice tests. Become familiar with the format of multiple-choice questions. Use the CNOR practice tests as a method of improving your knowledge and identifying areas for further study.

When answering practice questions, consider the following as methods to avoid making testing errors:

- Read each question carefully. Errors are made when you do not read the question carefully and completely. Look for and identify the important points involved with the question. Read each option carefully, noting which option most closely matches the intent of the question. Eliminate the options that are not correct and choose the best response that addresses the question being asked.

- Assume that all of the information you need is presented in the test question. The stem of a multiple-choice test question should contain all of the information that is necessary for the test taker to answer the question. When you read the question, avoid the common pitfall of "reading into" the question. Doing this may only confuse you. If certain patient characteristics, such as age, diagnosis, clinical setting, or other related information, are important to know to answer the question, it will be provided. Otherwise, answer the question from the perspective of the most common situation.

- Identify content areas where your knowledge base is weak. Use the practice test as an opportunity to evaluate your current knowledge of perioperative nursing. When you answer questions incorrectly, use the opportunity to learn the reasons for the incorrect answers. Ask yourself, "Why was my choice wrong?" The best way to learn the content is to understand the underlying rationale for the correct as well as the incorrect answers.

- Understand the basic intent of the test question. One of the most common errors that test takers make is not understanding the intent of the question. Is the question asking for you to make a decision about identifying a priority, a sequence of events, or an important patient presentation? Often in these types of questions, all of the options are plausible for the situation, but the correct answer is the one that is most important, has the highest priority, or is the first action to be taken. Look for the guiding words that give you the direction or emphasis to take.

Day-of-Test Checklist

Within 24 hours before the examination, you should:

- Avoid engaging in any known stressful events. Many of us know what events tend to cause us stress. If at all possible, try to avoid engaging in or attending events that are known stressors just before taking the examination. Practice using relaxation methods to create a calm mental perspective about the test. This will enable you to think clearly and problem solve the questions.

- Obtain sufficient rest and sleep. Fatigue and lethargy will only inhibit your thinking and problem-solving abilities. Engage in any sleep rituals that tend to promote your sleeping ability.

- Limit use of any stimulants, including coffee. Stimulants will affect your ability to receive sufficient rest and sleep. Avoid taking any stimulants, including coffee, late in the day and before bedtime the night before the test.

- Arrive at the testing center at least 30 minutes before your test appointment. If you are unsure of the exact location of the test center, it is strongly suggested that you locate the test center ahead of time. Determine how long it will take you to drive there or go by public transportation, if applicable, by following the route before the day of your test. The test center can provide you with directions if you need them or go online and print out directions. Unforeseen and uncontrollable events, such as accidents or inclement weather, can cause delays in your travel time. It is far better to arrive early than to be late and miss your appointment.

- Limit the personal items you bring with you. You will not be permitted to take handbags, wallets, books, watches. cellular phones, laptops, or any other personal belongings into the testing room. The test center has lockers where you can store any items you bring. The proctor will provide you with scrap paper. There is no space at the test center for family members or friends to accompany you to your testing appointment.

- Make sure that you bring one form of identification with you to the test center. It must be current, government-issued photo identification, such as a driver's license or a passport, with a signature. Be sure your identification matches exactly the name on your Authorization to Test letter.

After the Examination

Try to avoid "second guessing." While it is common practice to "relive" the test experience, try not to second guess the responses you gave to each test question. Without the content of the question directly in front of you, it is too easy to "conclude" you may have answered incorrectly.

Do not share information about the test or test questions. Remember that you have signed a pledge to keep the contents of the CNOR certification examination confidential. Sharing information about the test or discussing specific questions about the test with colleagues or other test takers violates this confidentiality pledge. In addition, multiple forms of the examination are being administered so it is highly likely that the questions you saw on your test will not be the exact same questions another test taker saw.

Summary

Success occurs when you have made a detailed plan for preparing for the examination and have stuck to it! Essential components of success include:

- Identifying knowledge areas for review.
- Understanding the testing process.
- Being confident that your study habits have prepared you to be successful.

Self-Assessment for the CNOR Exam

CCI wants to help prepare you for success in seeking the professional credential for perioperative registered nurses (CNOR). The following self-assessment tool may be used to determine readiness for taking the exam, identify areas of strength and needed improvement, and aid in the development of a test preparation plan.

1. Have I met the criteria for eligibility to take the exam?
   Yes No
   - ☐ ☐ Have a current unrestricted RN license.
   - ☐ ☐ Be currently working full-time or part-time in perioperative nursing in the area of nursing education, administration, research, or clinical practice.
   - ☐ ☐ Have completed a minimum of 2 years and 2,400 hours of experience in perioperative nursing, with a minimum of 50% (1,200 hours) in the intraoperative setting.

> *Please check the CCI website (www.cc-institute.org) for the most current eligibility requirements. CCI reserves the right to change eligibility requirements at any time.*

2. Does my day-to-day practice involve a variety of surgical procedures, specialties, and patient age groups, or is my role restricted to one or two specialties or age groups?

My current practice involves
the following types of cases:

I will need additional exposure/information
on the following types of cases:

____

____

____

____

____

3. Do I perform my own preoperative assessment, or do I mostly rely on documentation from admitting personnel in developing my plan of care?

4. Do I know the action, dose, side effects, and contraindications for the medications my patient is taking pre-procedure?
    □ Yes   □ No

5. Do I know the action, dose, route, side effects, and contraindications for the medications that are administered during the intraoperative period?
    □ Yes   □ No

6. Do I have access to central processing personnel and resources?
    □ Yes   □ No

7. Do I participate in hand-offs to PACU nurses, or does someone else give report to the RN?

8. Is my facility current on Joint Commission, CMS, and other regulatory standards?
    □ Yes   □ No

9. Are Association of periOperative Registered Nurses (AORN) standards and recommended practices cited in my facility's policies and procedures?
    □ Yes   □ No

10. Do I incorporate the most current AORN standards and recommended practices into my practice?
    □ Yes   □ No

11. Are my facility's policies and procedures updated to reflect current best practice?
    □ Yes   □ No

12. Does my facility library/unit manager/educator have access to current reference and resource materials (e.g., *Perioperative Standards and Recommended Practices, Alexander's Care of the Patient in Surgery, Berry and Kohn's Operating Room Technique,* and/or *Competency for Safe Patient Care During Operative and Invasive Procedures*)?
    □ Yes   □ No

13. Have I provided myself with adequate time to study (typically 3 months) prior to taking the exam?
    □ Yes   □ No

14. Have I reviewed CCI's handbook (found at www.cc-institute.org) to familiarize myself with the testing process?
    □ Yes   □ No

15. Do I have a mentor or resource person who understands the certification process?
    □ Yes Person's name: _______________________________   □ No
           Contact info: _______________________________

16. Does my facility have a CCI Champion? (go to www.cc-institute.org for a list of Champions)
    □ Yes   Champion's name: _______________________________   □ No

17. I have identified and put a plan in place to address barriers to preparation for the exam:
    □ Cost of exam
    □ Cost of study materials
    □ Facility support/reward/recognition
    □ Time
    □ Testing anxiety

Step Back

Critically analyze the results of your self-assessment. Numerous "no" answers, limited exposure to all components of perioperative nursing (pre-, intra-, and postoperative), and/or specialization to specific types of patients or procedures does not mean you cannot be successful on the exam, but it does suggest participating in additional learning opportunities to address identified deficits.

Learning Needs Assessment

The CNOR exam is based on the following domains, or major topics. The following tool can be used to evaluate your knowledge of items found on the CNOR examination. Together with the self-assessment, this tool provides a baseline for determining preparation needs. For each domain, score your current knowledge based on the following key:

1 — Very Certain: I know this content area well and believe that my work experiences have fully prepared me. I am comfortable with current practices and believe I am up-to-date with new developments and advances.

2 — Certain: I am reasonably comfortable with this content area and believe that my work experiences have prepared me fairly well.

3 — Undecided: I have some knowledge and some experience in this area, but there may be a few content areas where I am not as strong or for which my work experiences have not fully prepared me.

4 — Uncertain: I am aware that I have some knowledge deficits and/or a lack of work experience in this content area. I will need to engage in some study or other remediation to be comfortable with this content area.

5 — Very Uncertain: I am aware that I have many knowledge deficits and/or lack work experiences in this content area. This is an area of weakness for me and one that will require me to remediate before taking the examination.

Match the percentage of questions in the domain and the areas scored 3, 4, or 5 to help determine what content will need the most review.

Domain	My level of competency	Percentage of questions on the exam
1. Preoperative Assessment and Diagnosis		14%
2. Identify Expected Outcomes and Develop an Individualized Plan of Care		9%
3. Intraoperative Activities		31%
4. Communication		9%
5. Transfer of Care		5%
6. Cleaning, Disinfecting, Packaging, Sterilizing, Transporting, and Storing Instruments and Supplies		12%
7. Emergency Situations		8%
8. Management of Personnel, Services, and Materials		6%
9. Professional Accountability		6%

NOTES

CHAPTER 1:
Preoperative Patient Assessment and Diagnosis

> **Test Specifications:**
> *14% of CNOR test questions are based on Preoperative Patient Assessment and Diagnosis.*

Introduction

Patient assessment is the cornerstone of all nursing practice. It is the first item listed in the nursing process, and although perioperative nurses may conduct a more focused assessment than a med-surg or critical care nurse, the more information we gather, the better able we will be to identify special needs (diagnosis), determine our next steps (plan of care), and anticipate what we would like to happen (expected outcomes). The next two chapters provide opportunities to apply what we know to common perioperative situations. A patient-centered approach is utilized for several reasons:

1. The Institute of Medicine has identified this as one of six needed health care competencies (IOM, 2001).

2. Utilizing a patient-centered approach helps keep the focus on patient care, rather than on what an individual nurse would do based on a facility's policies and procedures.

Although checklists and preference cards are useful in helping us organize and complete tasks in the OR, these tools are not as beneficial in developing a plan of care from the patient's perspective. A concept or mind map (see sample on the following page) is an organizational tool that allows us to look at the connection between our patients' needs and how we meet those needs. It also is a good reminder that events do not necessarily occur in order, and certainly not in isolation; multiple things can and do happen at the same time, and one event can have an impact on many other systems. The concept map will encourage us to view the big picture, ask questions about our patients, and allow us to appreciate the interrelatedness of data obtained from our patient assessment and our plan of care.

There is no one "correct" way to develop a concept map; the samples on the CD that came with this *Guide* are examples only and are to be used to help get you started. Feel free to develop your own map. It is more important to develop a tool that you can use and that makes sense to you than to strictly follow the examples. Although they may be arranged differently, you will find that the main components of your map will be the same as those found in the learning activities.

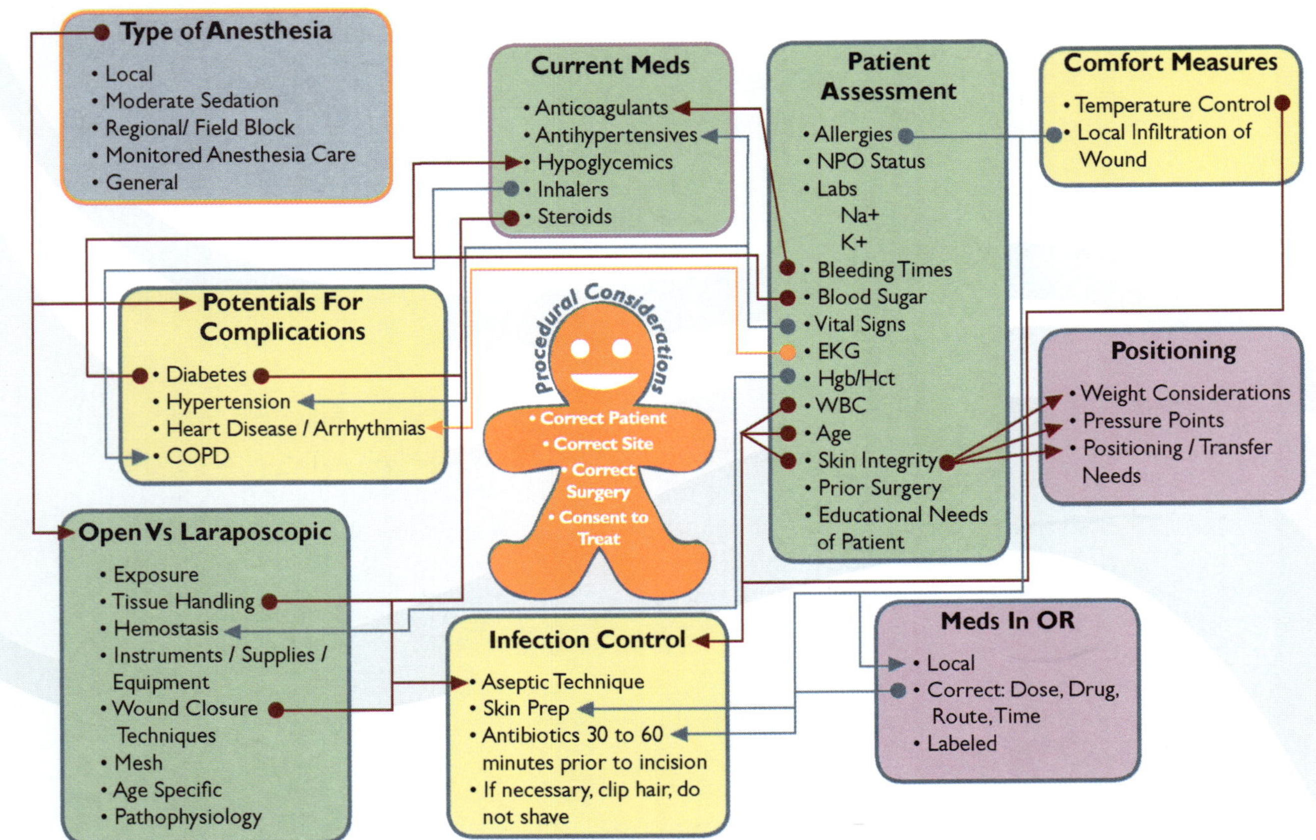

Concept Map - Inguinal Hernia Repair, *J. Mower*

Case Study

To encourage continuity in learning activities between pre-, intra-, and postoperative patient care, a case study approach will be presented in Chapters 1, 2, 3, 5, and 8. Our imaginary patient will guide us through critical thinking exercises that can be applied to any patient, of any age, and for any procedure. Templates for forms are included on the CD for you to make multiple copies as you wish in developing your own plans of care.

The case study for this *Guide* is presented on the following two pages. Case study activities presented in this and later chapters appear in a box with an orange border as shown on the next page.

Case Study

Note: *This case study will be used for activities in Chapters 1, 2, 3, 5, and 8.*

Your first patient of the day is Mrs. M., who is scheduled for a laparoscopic chole-cystectomy at 0730. You assist your scrub technologist in opening the room, and then go to AM Admissions to meet your patient. After reviewing Mrs. M.'s medical record and conducting your preoperative interview, you have obtained the following information:

Chief Complaint:
Cholecystitis, cholelithiasis
Nausea and vomiting (NV) and Right Upper Quadrant (RUQ) pain X 1 week; worsens after eating, especially with fatty foods. Ultrasound confirms diagnosis with report of multiple small stones in gall bladder.

Past Medical History:
Diabetes mellitus type II (Non-Insulin Dependent Diabetic Mellitus [NIDDM]), controlled with oral meds
Hypertensive, controlled with diuretic
Height 5'2"; 240 pounds. States "I know I should exercise, but it's hard because my knees hurt so bad. Plus, I get so hot I think I'm going to faint."
Surgeries: Carpal tunnel release right wrist, 2002, IV regional
                    Cesarean section X 2, 1980 and 1982, spinal anesthetic

Family History:
Father — deceased at age 56, myocardial infarction (MI)
Mother — living, fair health, diabetic and hypertensive
Brothers — X 2, fair health, both are diabetic
Significant for maternal grandmother dying during surgery to remove gallbladder, 1954. Patient states ,"I'm really worried that the same thing is going to happen to me."

Social:
Married, 3 children. Works as administrative assistant for CNO for large medical center. Smokes 1 pack per day (ppd) X 20 years. Drinks 1 glass of wine/day.

Allergies:
Penicillin (PCN) — hives, swelling of face and hands
Multiple fruits (strawberries, kiwi, bananas) — hives
Face broke out and became short of breath after last visit to dentist

Continued on following page.

Case Study, *continued*

Medications:

Glucophage — 500 mg twice a day

Hydrochlorothiazide — 25 mg every day

Multivitamin — 1 every day

Gingko Biloba — 60 mg every day

Naproxen — 220 mg twice a day

Took usual meds this morning with sip of water; otherwise has been NPO since midnight.

Physical Exam:

54-year-old woman in moderate distress. Abdomen soft, obese. Guards RUQ. Last emesis 2 hours ago; approximately "½ cup" (120 ml) of bile.

Vital signs

BP — 144/90 mmHg

P — 50 bpm

Pulse ox — 95% on room air

T (TM) — 99.2° F

R — 16/min

Diagnostic Tests and Lab Values:

Hematology	*Reference range*
WBCs — 12,000/mm^3	5,000-10,000/mm^3
RBCs — 4.5 x 10^{12}/mm^3	4.2-5.4 x 10^{12}/mm^3
Hemoglobin — 15.4 g/dl	12.0-16.0 g/dl
Hematocrit — 44.0%	38-47%
HgbA1c — 8.1%	less than 7%
Na+ — 137 mEq/L	136-145 mEq/L
K+ — 3.0 mEq/L	3.5-5.0 mEq/L
CO_2 — 25 mEq/L	23-29 mEq/L
Cl- — 101 mEq/L	98-107 mEq/L
Blood glucose — 102 mg/dl	74-100 mg/dl
Ca++ — 10.1 mg.dl	8.6-10.2 mg/dl
BUN — 17 mg/dl	8-23 mg/dl
Creatinine — 0.9 mg/dl	0.8-1.3 mg/dl

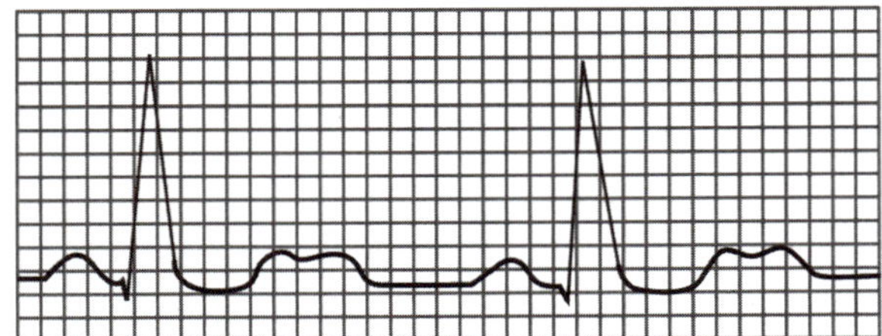

Patient has an IV in her left hand with Lactated Ringers 1,000 ml infusing at 125 ml/hour. She is wearing sequential compression stockings.

Module 1: Assess the Health Status of the Patient

Patient assessment requires collecting data from a variety of sources and incorporating that information with physical and psychosocial findings to develop nursing diagnoses, which will drive the plan of care. Thorough documentation of findings will help prevent duplication or omission of data.

Competency Outcomes

To successfully complete the activities in this module, you will need to be able to:

1. Differentiate normal from abnormal anatomy and physiology based on age-related factors.
2. Integrate components of relevant pathophysiologic processes (concurrent disease processes, inflammatory/immune responses, etc.) into a surgical patient plan of care.
3. Collect, analyze, and prioritize patient data (allergies, lab values, EKG, arterial blood gas results, other medical conditions, previous relevant surgical history, NPO status) from a variety of sources (chart review, patient/family interview, consultation with other health care team members).
4. Conduct an individualized physical assessment.
5. Select nursing diagnoses based on data collected during the preoperative assessment period.
6. Demonstrate cultural competence in assessing needs for a diverse patient population.
7. Provide for continuity in patient care by documenting the preoperative assessment.

Recommended Readings

Perioperative Standards and Recommended Practices (2013), Section 1: Standards of perioperative nursing practice; Recommended practices for minimally invasive surgery.

Alexander's Care of the Patient in Surgery. (2011, 14th ed.), Chapter 1: Concepts basic to perioperative nursing; Unit II: Surgical interventions.

Berry and Kohn's Operating Room Technique. (2013, 12th ed.), Chapter 2: Foundations of perioperative patient care standards; Chapter 7: The patient: The reason for your existence; Chapter 9: Perioperative geriatrics; Chapter 11: Ambulatory surgery centers and alternative surgical locations; Chapter 21: Preoperative preparation of the patient; Chapter 25: Coordinated roles of the scrub person and the circulating nurse.

Competency for Safe Patient Care During Operative and Invasive Procedures. (2009), Chapter 5: Preparation of the patient for the procedure.

Key Words

Age specific, assessment, diagnostic studies, laboratory results, nursing diagnosis, nursing process, patient education, *Perioperative Nursing Data Set* (PNDS), physical assessment, preoperative testing

Patient Assessment

Importance of Assessment

The first step in the nursing process, assessment, is performed throughout the patient's entire health care experience. The initial assessment identifies baseline values through information provided by the patient, family and guardians, significant others, the medical record, lab work, and other health care providers. This information will be used to formulate perioperative nursing diagnoses and the patient's plan of care, reinforcing the need to both obtain and accurately interpret data.

Components of the Patient Assessment

Rather than a head-to-toe or complete review of systems, perioperative nurses typically perform a more focused patient assessment based on data found in the history and physical and patient interview that are directly applicable to the proposed operative or invasive procedure.

Documentation of Assessment Findings

Whether electronic or paper, results of the assessment must be noted to ensure continuity of care. Many facilities have preprinted forms, which serve as excellent reminders of components that need to be included in the assessment and help to decrease errors or omissions in the assessment process. Although checklists and boxes are convenient and efficient, all records should have the capability of allowing the nurse to add additional information to reflect a patient's individual needs, as this information is especially important in developing a plan of care. Patients may reveal important information to the nurse that they did not relay to other health care providers; this could affect the surgical procedure or the type of anesthesia planned. Documentation of the patient's assessment should include findings of the focused exam and patient interview.

Activity — Fill in the Blank

1. Sources of data used in developing the plan of care include: *pt, family, gaurdians medical record labs, ECG other staff*

2. Perioperative nurses are more likely to perform a *focused* patient assessment.

3. The purpose of documenting assessment findings is to ensure *continuity of care* and should include results of *physical exam* and *interview*.

"Go To" Case Study Activity
Draw Your Own Concept Map

Go to the Concept Map file on the CD that came with this *Guide*. Following the instructions on the CD, and using the patient information on pages 35-36, begin drawing your concept map that organizes the data you will need to develop your surgical plan of care. The steps involved are repeated here for your convenience.

Put your patient's name, preoperative diagnosis, and proposed procedure in the center of the map.

Make a list of all the data you feel you will need to address in your plan of care.

Identify Mrs. M.'s "major problems." Some of these are typical for every surgery (e.g., infection, pain, anxiety), while others will be specific for Mrs. M. Eventually these will turn into nursing diagnoses; for now, just label them with whatever terms you're comfortable using. Put each "major problem" into its own box.

Arrange the assessment data from your list under their corresponding "major problems" boxes. The same data may be used in multiple boxes.

What critical information needs to be communicated to the following health care team members?

Anesthesia provider: *[handwritten: → feeling "faint → long term?) ↓K+ (EKG c̄ U wave flattened T), risk for MH (from mom died in sx), PCN + ? latex allergy (Dentist, kiwi, bananas) ⊕ NPO, glucophage (need BG)]*

Surgeon: *[handwritten: ↓K+, PCN + ? latex, ? MH, ? poss adverse reaction btwn glucophage + contrast (lactic acidosis → rare) hold glucophage/metformin x 48° to prevent issues]*

Scrub person: *[handwritten: Need longer inst., poss latex allergy]*

PACU: *[handwritten: PCN + ? latex allergy, poss. MH, BG]*

Activity — Matching

From the list of patient assessment data below, write the letter of its corresponding perioperative nursing intervention(s) on the right. (Note: some items will have multiple answers.)

Assessment Data:

Identification of patient _C, H_

Baseline vital signs (temperature, pulse, respirations, blood pressure, pulse oximetry reading, and pain assessment) _E, F, I, J_

Height and weight _A, C, D, E, G_

Known medical conditions _A, B, C, D, E, F, G, I, J_

Prescription and over-the-counter medications, supplements including herbal preparations taken on a routine basis, and last medication administration _B, C, J_

Allergies or sensitivities, including latex and food _B, C, F, J_

NPO status _B, F_

Previous surgical history, including asking about metal implants and untoward reactions to anesthesia _A–J_

Skin condition _A–E, G, J_

Level of consciousness _B, D, F, H_

Emotional status _B, C, H_

Risk for falling _B, C, D_

Any history of drug or alcohol abuse _B, C, E_

Smoking history (packs per day and pack years) _B, E, F_

Signs of physical or emotional abuse _B, G_

Diagnostic test results _A–C, E–G, J_

Diversity and cultural needs _B, H_

Knowledge deficits related to surgery/recovery _B, E, H_

Intervention:

A. Positioning

B. Patient education/communication

C. Medication and solution administration

D. Moving/transfer

E. Infection prevention

F. Adequate airway/oxygen exchange

G. Maintenance of skin integrity

H. Preventing wrong site, wrong patient, wrong procedure

I. Normothermia

J. Adequate tissue perfusion

"Go To" Activity — Skill Building

Spend a morning with the A.M. admission nurse in your facility. Observe interview and assessment techniques. How best can you effectively and efficiently integrate the information obtained in the preoperative area to your plan of care for the OR?

"Go To" Activity — Check It Out!

On the CD, go to Question #6, NPO Status, and Question #10, Hyperglycemia, under the Perioperative question of the week tab for additional critical-thinking questions.

"Go To" Activity — Skill Building

Compare your facility's policy and procedure on length of time for preoperative fasting with the American Society of Anesthesiologists' recommended guidelines. How do they differ?

Additional Readings/Resources

Kittelson, K.A. (2009). Glycemic control: A literature review with implications for perioperative nursing practice. *AORN Journal, 90*(5), 714-728. BONUS: Examination questions.

Peterson, C. (2010). Requirement for a history and physical examination before minor surgery. *AORN Journal, 92*(5), 586-587.

Module 2: Review of Preoperative Medications

Obtaining a detailed history of current medications and allergies is an excellent way to further understand a patient's overall state of health. Evaluating current medication information serves multiple purposes. It identifies allergies; concurrent disease processes and the severity of the condition; the effectiveness of the drug in treating the condition; the patient's knowledge of pharmacology related to his/her medications; and the history of compliance with a drug regimen (which may serve as a predictor for successfully following postoperative instructions). In addition, potential adverse effects and drug interactions between home, perioperative, and discharge medications can be identified early and thereby avoided.

Competency Outcomes

To successfully complete the activities in this module, you will need to be able to:

1. Reconcile current medications (preoperative medications, current prescription drugs, over-the-counter medications, alternative and herbal supplements, and medical marijuana) and alcohol and recreational drug consumption with patient's condition and proposed surgical procedure.
2. Identify possible adverse effects of patient's daily meds on the surgical procedure.

Recommended Readings

Perioperative Standards and Recommended Practices (2013), Recommended practices: Medication safety.

Alexander's Care of the Patient in Surgery. (2011, 14th ed.), Chapter 2: Patient safety and risk management; Chapter 29: Integrated health practices: Complementary and alternative therapies.

Berry and Kohn's Operating Room Technique. (2013, 12th ed.), Chapter 2: Foundations of perioperative patient care standards; Chapter 11: Ambulatory surgery centers and alternative surgical locations; Chapter 21: Preoperative preparation of the patient; Chapter 23: Surgical pharmacology, pp. 420-421.

Competency for Safe Patient Care During Operative and Invasive Procedures. (2009), Chapter 5: Preparation of the patient for the procedure; Chapter 12: Administer drugs and solutions.

Key Words

Complementary/alternative medicine (CAM), allergies, herbs, medication reconciliation, patient/family education, pharmacology, side effects

---

Case Study Activity — Matching

Match Mrs. M.'s current medications to their action from the list at the right.

Glucophage __C__

Hydrochlorothiazide __A__

Gingko Biloba __D__

Naproxen __B__

A. diuretic; inhibits sodium reabsorption

B. nonsteroidal anti-inflammatory

C. decreases hepatic glucose production, increases insulin sensitivity

D. memory enhancer (controversial)

Case Study Activity — Critical Thinking

How does Mrs. M.'s allergy to penicillin affect the choice of prophylactic antibiotic?

Limits choice of ABT. & Ancef.

Which of Mrs. M.'s home medications could influence the surgical procedure? Why?

Naproxen + Gingko Biloba together ↑ risk for bleeding

Additional Readings/Resources

American Society of Anesthesiologists (n.d.). Herbal supplements and anesthesia. Retrieved Jan. 31, 2013, from http://www.lifelinetomodernmedicine.com/sitecore/content/Home.aspx. Bonus: Includes a video.

Ang-Lee, M.K., Moss, J., & Yuan, C-S. (2001). Herbal medicines and perioperative care. *Journal of the American Medical Association, 286*, 208-216. Retrieved Jan. 31, 2013, from http://jama.ama-assn.org/content/286/2/208.full.pdf+html

Chard, R. (2009). Medication reconciliation across the continuum of care. *AORN Journal, 92*(4), 470-471.

Module 3: Initiation of the Universal Protocol

The Universal Protocol was initiated by The Joint Commission to prevent wrong site, wrong procedure, and wrong person surgery. A standardized checklist that is consistently initiated and followed has been found to help decrease surgical errors.

Competency Outcomes

To successfully complete the activities in this module, you will need to be able to:

1. Apply components of the Universal Protocol.
2. Identify AORN standards and recommended practices that help to prevent adverse outcomes.

Recommended Readings

Alexander's Care of the Patient in Surgery. (2011, 14th ed.), Chapter 2: Patient safety and risk management; Chapter 11: Surgery of the liver, biliary tract, pancreas, and spleen.

Berry and Kohn's Operating Room Technique. (2013, 12th ed.), Chapter 2: Foundations of perioperative patient care standards; Chapter 3: Legal, regulatory, and ethical issues.

Competency for Safe Patient Care During Operative and Invasive Procedures. (2009), Chapter 6: Transfer the patient.

Key Words

The Joint Commission (TJC), preoperative verification, site marking, wrong site, wrong procedure, wrong person

Activity — Fill in the Blank

Preoperative verification to prevent wrong __*patient*__, __*site*__, or __*procedure*__ includes ensuring that all relevant documents are available prior to the procedure.

What documents can be used to verify the patient's procedure?

consent (sx)   *bld tx consent*

H+P   *sx sched*   *labs*

consent (anes)   *imaging*

What components of the Universal Protocol are incorporated in the preoperative area?

1. *Pt verification using 2 identifiers*

2. *Marking site*

Activity — Critical Thinking

For the following never events, identify the corresponding AORN standard or recommended practices that address it. There may be multiple correct answers.

Answer:

1. Surgery performed on the wrong body part, the wrong patient, or the wrong procedure.

Position statement on preventing wrong-site, wrong pt, wrong procedure events

2. Unintended retention of a foreign object in a patient after surgery or other procedure.

Recommended practices: Prevention of Retained surgical items

3. Patient death or serious disability associated with a medication error.

Recom. practices: medication safety

4. Patient death or serious disability associated with a burn incurred from any source.

R.P: Laser safety, electrosurgery, preoperative pt skin asepsis

5. Hospital acquired pressure ulcers.

R.P: positioning the pt.

6. Deep vein thrombosis.

R.P.: Prevention of DVT

7. Hospital acquired surgical site infections.

R.P: hand hygiene, Sterile technique, traffic patterns, environmental cleaning, prevention of transmissable infections, prevention of hypothermia, preop pt skin asepsis, + sterilization

Activity — Mark the Site

Based on The Joint Commission guidelines, mark the torso illustration for a right inguinal hernia repair.

Additional Readings/ Resources

Conrardy, J.A., Brenek, B., & Myers, S. (2010). Determining the state of knowledge for implementing the Universal Protocol recommendations: An integrative review of the literature. *AORN Journal, 92*(2), 194-207.

Guglielmi, C. (2010). Table talk: Strategies for preventing wrong site, wrong procedure, and wrong patient surgery. *AORN Journal, 92*(1), 22-27.

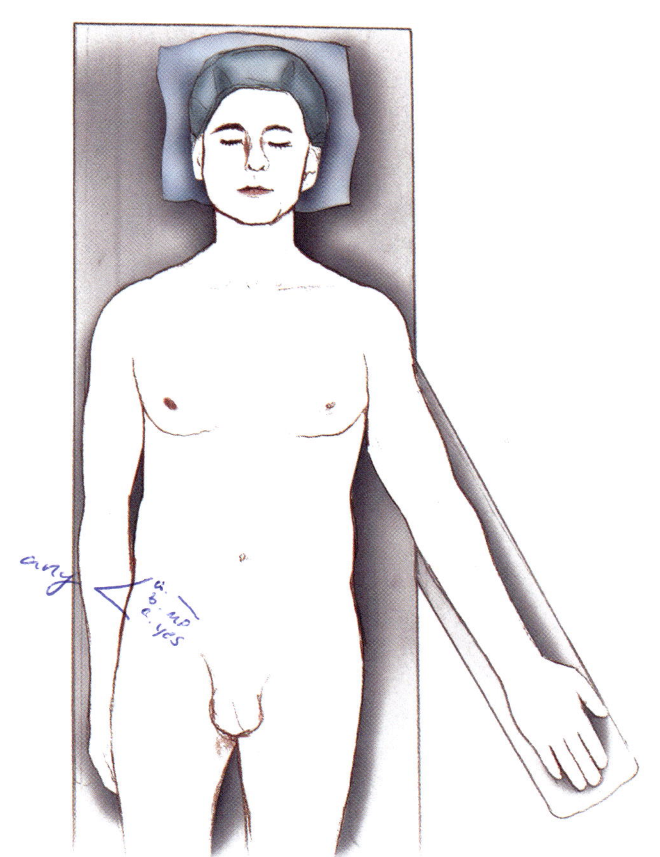

Module 4: Obtaining Surgical Consent

Informed consent is a contract between the patient and the health care practitioner performing the operation or invasive procedure. The reason for the procedure and its risks, benefits, complications, and alternatives must be explained in terms the patient can understand. The consent serves as one of the major documents on which the perioperative nurse relies when developing a plan of care.

Competency Outcomes

To successfully complete the activities in this module, you will need to be able to:

1. Identify components of a surgical consent.
2. Define "informed consent."
3. Outline steps for obtaining consent.

Recommended Readings

Alexander's Care of the Patient in Surgery. (2011, 14th ed.), Chapter 2: Patient safety and risk management.

Berry and Kohn's Operating Room Technique. (2013, 12th ed.), Chapter 3: Legal, regulatory, and ethical issues.

Key Words

Alternatives, autonomy, benefits, complications, informed consent, patient rights, privacy, respect, risk, teaching back

Activity — Fill in the Blank

The surgeon or practitioner performing the procedure is responsible for informing the patient about the proposed procedure in terms that he or she can understand.

It is the _____Surgeon_____'s responsibility to obtain informed consent.

Activity — Critical Thinking

How does obtaining surgical consent for a child differ from that of an adult?

> **"Go To" Activity — Check It Out!**
>
> On the CD, go to Question #28, Informed consent and minors, under the Perioperative question of the week tab for an additional critical-thinking question.

Case Study Activity — Consent

Mrs. M.'s consent states that she is scheduled for a laparoscopic cholecystectomy, possible open, with cholangiograms.

1. How will you evaluate Mrs. M.'s understanding of the proposed procedure?

   Open ended questions

2. What puts Mrs. M. at risk for converting to an open procedure?

   Wt, prev. sp

"Go To" Activity — Skill Building

Obtain a consent form from your facility. Compare it with the documentation typically included on an informed consent:

- Name of patient
- Name of facility where procedure will be performed
- Surgical procedure
- Site/side as applicable
- Benefits, risks, alternatives
- Person(s) performing the procedure
- Statement that procedure was explained to the patient/legal guardian
- Signature of the patient or legal guardian
- Signature of the surgeon
- Signature of witness
- Date and time consent is obtained
- Additional permissions requested (for example, blood transfusions, presence of visitors/students, photographs)

Additional Readings/Resources

Burlingame, B. (2009). Length of time a signed informed consent is valid. *AORN Journal, 90*(3), 446-447.

Peterson, C. (2010). Responsibility for obtaining the surgical informed consent. In Clinical issues, *AORN Journal, 92*(5), 585-586.

Module 5: Ensuring Patients' Rights By Providing Information on Advance Directives, Do-Not-Resuscitate

Patients undergoing an operative or invasive procedure have the same rights in determining the course of their care as any other patient. Clear communication between the patient and the surgical team is even more important, as the nature of the care provided during a procedure may mimic a resuscitative event.

Competency Outcomes

To successfully complete the activities in this module, you will need to be able to:

1. Define the terms "advance directive" and "do-not-resuscitate (DNR)."
2. Describe ramifications of a DNR for a surgical patient.
3. Describe methods for confirming advance directive status or DNR status.

Recommended Readings

Perioperative Standards and Recommended Practices (2013), Position statement: Perioperative care of patients with do-not-resuscitate orders; Perioperative explications, 1.4: The right to self-determination.

Alexander's Care of the Patient in Surgery. (2011, 14th ed.), Chapter 2: Patient safety and risk management.

Berry and Kohn's Operating Room Technique. (2013, 12th ed.), Chapter 3: Legal, regulatory, and ethical issues.

Key Words

Advance directive, do-not-resuscitate (DNR), Patient Self-Determination Act (PSDA)

Activity — True or False?

Under the Patient Self-Determination Act, patients have the legal right to accept or refuse medical treatment, including resuscitation, even if refusal will likely result in death.

TRUE __X__   FALSE ____

"Go To" Activity — Check It Out!

Go to Question #8, Patient rights and DNR, under the Perioperative question of the week tab on your CD for an additional critical-thinking question.

"Go To" Activity — Skill Building

What is your facility's policy on DNR for surgical patients? Do you have a separate form that must be filled out? If so, how many of the following choices does it include?
* suspension of DNR orders.
* continuation of DNR orders.
* limited resuscitation with procedure-directed orders.
* limited resuscitation with goal-directed orders.

Module 6: Pain Assessment

The importance of pain assessment is reflected by the fact that it is now being considered the "fifth vital sign." An initial baseline pain assessment obtained preoperatively is necessary as signs and symptoms of both acute and chronic pain may be masked by the medications given during the intraoperative period.

Competency Outcomes

To successfully complete the activities in this module, you will need to be able to:

1. Assess a patient for signs and symptoms of pain, taking into account variations related to age, gender, and culture.
2. Utilize a pain-rating scale in assessing a patient's level of pain.
3. Incorporate pain-relief interventions into a plan of care.

Recommended Readings

Alexander's Care of the Patient in Surgery. (2011, 14th ed.), Chapter 4: Anesthesia; Chapter 9: Postoperative patient care and pain management; Chapter 25: Pediatric surgery; Chapter 26: Geriatric surgery; Chapter 29: Integrated health practices: Complementary and alternative therapies.

Berry and Kohn's Operating Room Technique. (2013, 12th ed.), Chapter 8: Perioperative pediatrics; Chapter 30: Postoperative patient care.

Competency for Safe Patient Care During Operative and Invasive Procedures. (2009), Chapter 18: Facilitate care after the procedure; Chapter 36: Clinical aspects of operative pain.

Key Words

Analgesia, narcotics, nonsteroidal anti-inflammatories (NSAIDS), nonpharmacologic interventions, opioids, pain assessment, pain block, pain intensity scales, patient-controlled analgesia (PCA), pharmacology, regional anesthesia, self-report, signs, symptoms, The Joint Commission (TJC)

Activity — Matching

Match the most appropriate pain rating scale to the patient described below. (Answers may be used more than once.)

3-year-old girl ____

45-year-old man ____

23-year-old woman who does not speak English ____

A. 0-10 Numeric pain intensity scale

B. FACES Pain rating scale

C. Simple descriptive pain intensity scale

Case Study Activity — Pain Assessment

How can you incorporate components of Mrs. M.'s age, sex, ethnicity, and culture into her pain management plan? (Note: This same format may be utilized when developing any patient's pain treatment plan.)

Additional Readings/Resources

Trudeau, J.D., Lamb, E., Gowans, M., & Lauder, G. (2009). A prospective audit of post-operative pain control in pediatric patients. *AORN Journal, 90*(4), 531-542.
Note: This article provides a nice description of another pain rating tool, FLACC (Face, Legs, Activity, Cry, Consolability).

Module 7: Development of Nursing Diagnoses

A nursing diagnosis sorts assessment data into real or potential patient problems. Standardized terminology is used to "label" the problem, which enhances clear communication and documentation among members of the health care team. Nursing interventions specific to each diagnosis are then identified. Experience level determines the speed with which a practitioner moves through these steps.

Competency Outcomes

To successfully complete the activities in this module, you will need to be able to:

1. Identify common perioperative nursing diagnoses.
2. Formulate nursing diagnoses that are consistent with the patient's assessment data.

Recommended Readings

Alexander's Care of the Patient in Surgery. (2011, 14th ed.), Chapter 1: Concepts basic to perioperative nursing.

Berry and Kohn's Operating Room Technique. (2013, 12th ed.), Chapter 2: Foundations of perioperative patient care standards.

Competency for Safe Patient Care During Operative and Invasive Procedures. (2009), Chapter 2: Competency assessment.

Key Words

Diagnosis, medical diagnosis, nursing diagnosis, nursing process, *Perioperative Nursing Data Set* (PNDS)

Frequently Used Nursing Diagnoses

Acute pain	Nausea
Anxiety	Risk for aspiration
Chronic pain	Risk for deficient fluid volume
Deficient knowledge	Risk for electrolyte imbalance
Fear	Risk for imbalanced body temperature
Hyperthermia	Risk for imbalanced fluid volume
Hypothermia	Risk for impaired skin integrity
Imbalanced nutrition	Risk for infection
Impaired gas exchange	Risk for injury
Impaired transfer ability	Risk for latex allergy response
Ineffective breathing pattern	Risk for perioperative positioning injury
Ineffective health maintenance	Risk for peripheral neurovascular dysfunction

Source: AORN. (2011). *Perioperative Nursing Data Set* (3rd ed., p. 416). Denver: AORN, Inc.

"Go To" Case Study Activity — Nursing Diagnoses

From your interpretation of Mrs. M.'s assessment data, formulate nursing diagnoses to address each identified problem or potential problem. Write your nursing diagnoses in the boxes next to your "major problem" in your concept map on the CD. Not all of your "major problems" may have a corresponding nursing diagnosis.

Activity — Matching

Match the term with its definition.

Etiology ___B___

Nursing diagnosis ___F___

Nursing intervention ___D___

Problem ___E___

Sign ___A___

Symptom ___C___

A. Objective information obtained through the five senses

B. Cause of a disease supported by medical data

C. Subjective information obtained through what the patient tells you

D. Actions for which the perioperative nurse is accountable

E. Any condition that requires a nursing intervention

F. Identification of a real or potential patient problem or risk

Chapter Summary

The perioperative nurse's assessment of the surgical patient and formulation of nursing diagnoses are critical components of safe, efficient patient care. This information serves as the focal point for mapping the patient's perioperative experience.

Glossary

Advance directive — Legal document that allows the patient to provide instruction ahead of time on end-of-life care.

AORN standards and recommended practices — This term includes all sections of the *Perioperative Standards and Recommended Practices* published annually by AORN. The most current edition should be used at all times.

Assessment — Collecting data about a patient to determine the appropriate nursing diagnoses and expected outcomes. This includes patient's history and physical, vital signs, all aspects of presenting condition, and results of diagnostic tests. Assessment begins with data collection and ends with the formulation of nursing diagnoses. Assessment is ongoing during the perioperative period (i.e., includes preoperative, intraoperative, postoperative periods).

Association of periOperative Registered Nurses (AORN) — AORN is the professional organization of perioperative registered nurses that supports registered nurses in achieving optimal outcomes for patients undergoing operative and other invasive procedures. (www.aorn.org)

Community resources — Other agencies that the perioperative nurse may refer patients to for special needs (e.g., American Cancer Society, American Heart Association, home health care agencies, social services, organ procurement agencies).

Continuum of care — Care of patients undergoing operative or other invasive procedures from the time the decision to undergo surgery is made, through the intraoperative period, and for an undetermined postoperative period until the patient's health status is improved or a specified health goal is reached.

Cultural diversity — Variances in beliefs, actions, customs, and values between racial, ethnic, religious, or social groups.

Discharge planning — The process of assessing the needs of patients for postprocedure care; developing a coordinated and multidisciplinary plan to provide the care required (including patient and family education, available services, and referral agencies and support groups); and evaluating the plan. The process begins before or on admission to the health care facility.

Documentation — The written record of nursing care including patient assessment, the actions taken as a result of that assessment, the plan of care developed and implemented, and the results of those actions. Documentation serves as the main, retrievable communication tool for the health care team.

Family — For purposes of this guide, significant others and extended family are included in the term "family."

Health literacy — An integral part of patient education; the ability to read, understand, and follow instructions related to treatment.

Healthcare Insurance Portability and Accountability Act (HIPAA) — Legislation passed in 1996 that addresses various aspects of the use of patients' medical information, including confidentiality of patient information in the medical record, consent processes for access to patients' health information, and the right to sue the health plan provider.

Informed consent — The patient's right to make his or her own informed decisions based on information regarding treatment options, including the benefits, expected outcomes, risks, and potential complications; right to refuse treatment; and decisions regarding participation in research studies.

Interdisciplinary teams — Pharmacy, radiology, blood bank, laboratories, environmental services (i.e., housekeeping), biomedical engineering, etc.

Intervention (nursing) — Action taken based on patient assessment data with the intention of achieving one or more expected patient outcomes.

The Joint Commission — The independent accrediting organization that designates acceptable patient care and evaluates health care facilities' abilities to adhere to specific guidelines (e.g., documentation, processes, policies, and procedures). (www.jointcommission.org)

Medical diagnosis — A disease-based determination of a condition by a physician based on a review of patient signs and symptoms and diagnostic tests.

North American Nursing Diagnosis Association (NANDA) — The group that has developed a list of 155 accepted nursing diagnoses to ensure that documentation in all areas of nursing uses consistent, comparable terminology. (www.nanda.org) Also see *Perioperative Nursing Data Set.*

Nursing diagnosis — A statement derived by the registered nurse from evaluating the patient's responses to actual or potential problems/conditions. The nursing diagnosis provides the framework for nursing interventions which, when implemented, will enable the patient to attain specific desired outcomes. It is structured using standardized nursing nomenclature. Also see North American Nursing Diagnosis Association and *Perioperative Nursing Data Set.*

Nursing process — The critical thinking a nurse uses to assess the health status of patients, identify problems, develop and implement plans of care, and evaluate the patients' responses to that care.

Outcome criteria — Statements developed to identify the tasks or conditions to be implemented that will assist the patient in achieving the desired outcomes. Outcome criteria indicate an expected, measurable change in the patient's health status.

Patients' rights — The rights of every patient to seek and receive health care regardless of his or her race, religion, or culture and with respect for the individual's self-image, privacy, and other such considerations, in accordance with the Patients' Bill of Rights.

Perioperative period — Time commencing with the decision for surgical intervention and ending with a follow-up home/clinic evaluation. This period includes the preoperative, intraoperative, and postoperative phases.

Plan of care (or care plan) — A result of a systematic process of identifying expected patient outcomes and determining how to achieve them. It includes the list of interventions necessary to reach the expected outcome. The plan of care directs all nursing care activities related to each patient.

Perioperative Nursing Data Set (PNDS) — The perioperative nursing vocabulary guidebook that provides nursing diagnosis, nursing interventions, and patient outcomes statements specific to the perioperative environment.

Postoperative phase — Begins with admission to the postanesthesia care area and ends with the resolution of surgical sequelae.

Preoperative phase — Begins when the decision for surgical intervention is made and ends with the transfer of the patient to the operating room bed.

Regulatory standards — Federal, state, and local laws and regulations that govern practice.

Safe environment — The setting in which the physical and psychological aspects of the environment are controlled for the purpose of presenting the least possible hazard to the patient, staff members, and community.

Surgical intervention — The patient's experiences during the preoperative, intraoperative, and postoperative phases, including the technical aspects and anatomical approach.

Surgical procedure — The technical aspects and anatomical approach used during surgical intervention.

Teaching and learning theories and techniques — Those aids and methods that facilitate learning (e.g., audiovisual tools, return demonstration, and adult learning principles).

Time-out — As an integral component of The Joint Commission's Universal Protocol for Preventing Wrong Site, Wrong Procedure, and Wrong Person Surgery, a time-out surgical site verification must be conducted in the location where the procedure will be done, just before starting the procedure and, if possible, include active participation of the patient. It must involve the entire operative team, use active communication, be documented, and must include, at the least:
- Correct patient identity
- Correct side and site
- Agreement on the procedure to be done
- Correct patient position
- Availability of correct implants and any special equipment

References

AORN. (2011). *Perioperative Nursing Data Set* (3rd ed.). Denver: AORN, Inc.

AORN. (2013). *Perioperative Standards and Recommended Practices*. Denver: AORN, Inc.

Committee on Quality of Health Care in America, Institute of Medicine. (2001). *Crossing the Quality Chasm: A New Health System for the 21st Century*. Washington, D.C.: National Academies Press.

Guarisco, K. K. (2004). Managing do-not-resuscitate orders in the perianesthesia period. *Journal of Perianesthesia Nursing, 19*(5), 300-307.

The Joint Commission. (2013). Universal Protocol. Retrieved Jan. 31, 2013, from http://www.jointcommission.org/standards_information/up.aspx.

Rothrock, J.C. (Ed.). (2011). *Alexander's Care of the Patient in Surgery* (14th ed.). St. Louis: Mosby.

Phippen, M.L., Ulmer, B.C., & Wells, M.P. (2009). *Competency for Safe Patient Care During Operative and Invasive Procedures*. Denver: CCI.

Answers to Chapter 1 Activities

Module 1: Assess the health status of the patient — Pages 37-41

Activity — Fill in the Blank

1. Sources of data used in developing the plan of care include *patient, family, guardians, significant others, the medical record, lab work, and other health care providers.*

2. Perioperative nurses are more likely to perform a *focused* patient assessment.

3. The purpose of documenting assessment findings is to ensure *continuity of patient care* and should include results of *physical exam* and *patient interview.*

Case Study Activity — Draw Your Own Concept Map

Make a list of all the data you feel you will need to address in your plan of care.

Assessment data to be used in development of plan of care:

- Ultrasound shows multiple small stones
- Elevated temperature (99.2° F, 37.3° C)
- Elevated WBCs
- Pain
- Decreased mobility due to knee pain
- Nausea, vomiting
- EKG shows u wave, flattened T wave
- Potassium 3.0
- Diuretic
- Increased weight
- Surgical procedure; unexplained family death during surgery
- Smokes 1 pack per day
- Allergic to penicillin
- Food allergies (fruit)
- Fasting blood glucose 102 mg/dL; HgbA1C 8.2%
- Blood pressure 144/90 mmHg
- "Gets hot" when exercises
- Face "breaks out" at dentist

From the patient information noted above, begin drawing your concept map (on the CD) that identifies the data you will need to use in developing your surgical plan of care. Put your patient's name, preoperative diagnosis, and proposed procedure in the center of the map.

See concept maps on the the following pages for answers to the following related questions.

- Identify Mrs. M.'s "major problems," putting each into its own box.
- Arrange the data under their corresponding "major problems."

What critical information needs to be communicated to the following health care team members?

Anesthesia provider: ***Low K+, risk for MH, allergy to PCN, possible latex allergy, has been NPO and took Glucophage this am***

Surgeon: ***Low K+, risk for MH, possible latex allergy, possible adverse drug reaction between Glucophage and contrast medium***

Scrub person: ***Need for longer instrumentation, possible latex allergy***

PACU: ***Allergy to PCN, risk for MH, possible latex allergy***

Case Study Activity — Draw Your Own Concept Map, *continued*

SAMPLE Concept Map showing Mrs. M.'s major problems.

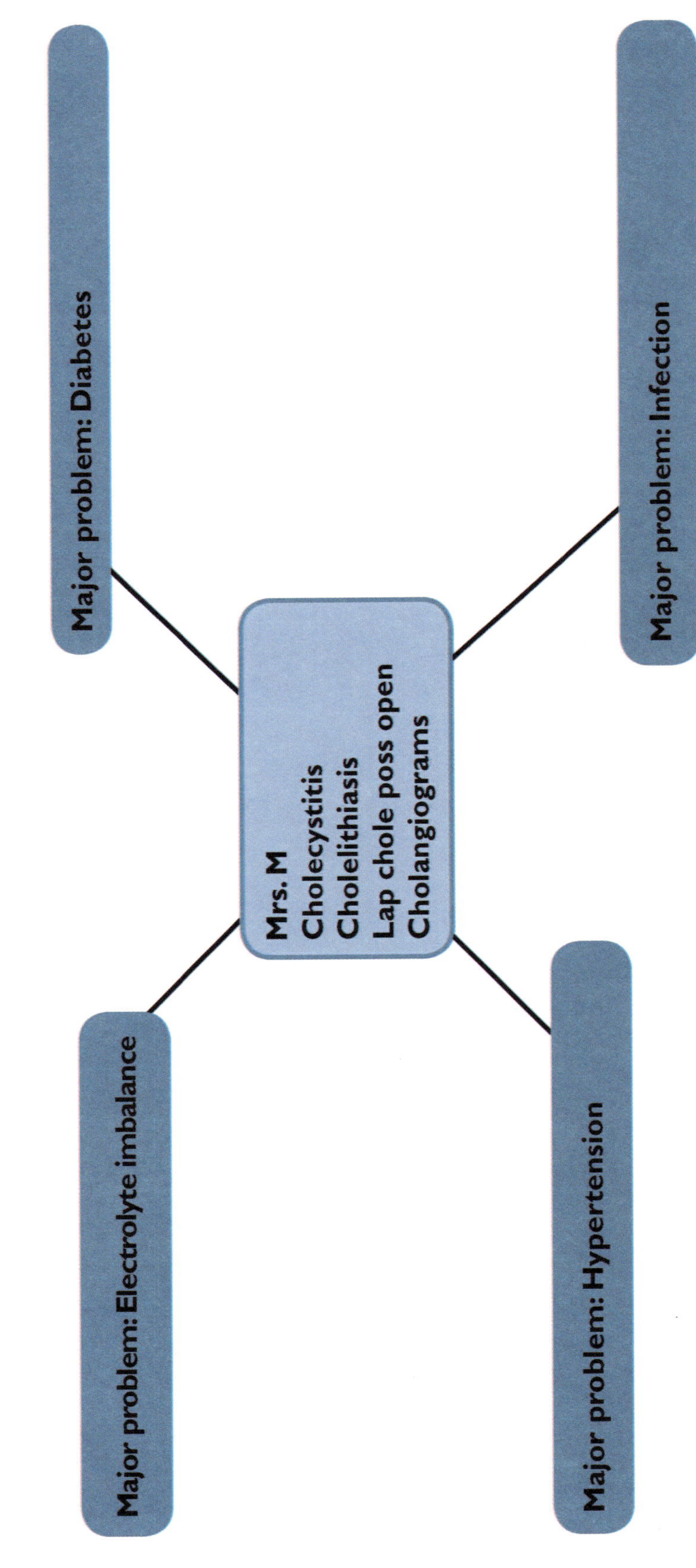

Case Study Activity — Draw Your Own Concept Map, *continued*

SAMPLE Concept Map showing the assessment data needed to develop a plan of care for Mrs. M.

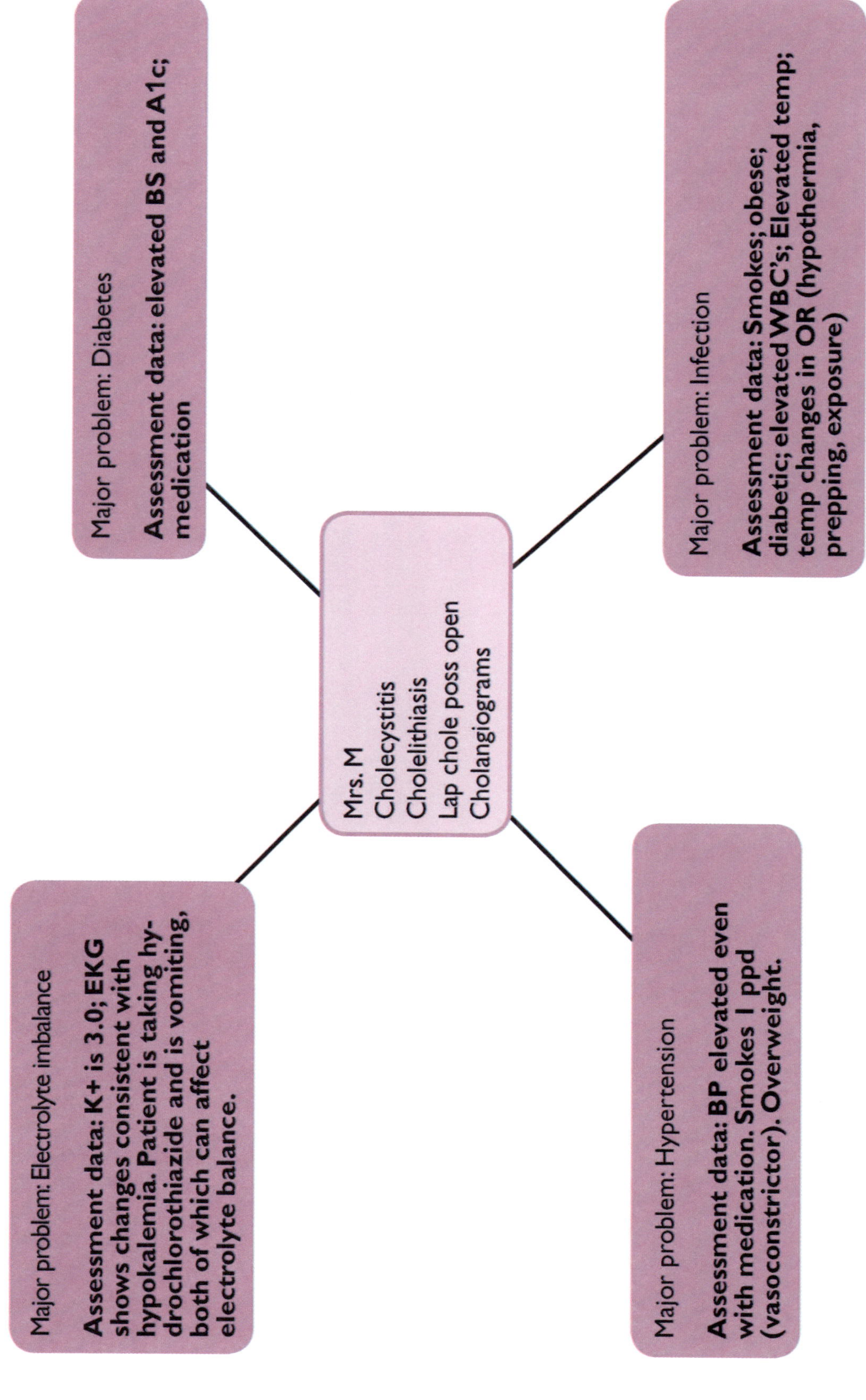

Activity — Matching

From the list of patient assessment data below, write the letter of its corresponding perioperative nursing intervention(s) on the right.

Assessment Data:

Identification of patient: *C, H*

Baseline vital signs (temperature, pulse, respirations, blood pressure, pulse oximetry reading, and pain assessment): *E, F, I, J*

Height and weight: *A, C, D, E, G*

Known medical conditions: *A, B, C, D, E, F, G, I, J*

Prescription and over-the-counter medications, supplements including herbal preparations taken on a routine basis, and last medication administration: *B, C, J*

Allergies or sensitivities, including latex and food: *B, C, F, J*

NPO status: *B, F*

Previous surgical history, including asking about metal implants and untoward reactions to anesthesia: *A, B, C, D, E, F, G, H, I, J*

Skin condition: *A, B, C, D, E, G, J*

Level of consciousness: *B, D, F, H*

Emotional status: *B, C, H*

Risk for falling: *B, C, D*

Any history of drug or alcohol abuse: *B, C, E*

Smoking history (packs per day and pack years): *B, E, F*

Signs of physical or emotional abuse: *B, G*

Diagnostic test results: *A, B, C, E, F, G, J*

Diversity and cultural needs: *B, H*

Knowledge deficits related to surgery/recovery: *B, E, H*

Interventions:

A. Positioning

B. Patient education/communication

C. Medication and solution administration

D. Moving/transfer

E. Infection prevention

F. Adequate airway/oxygen exchange

G. Maintenance of skin integrity

H. Preventing wrong site, wrong patient, wrong procedure

I. Normothermia

J. Adequate tissue perfusion

Source: Phippen, et al. (2009). *Competency for Safe Patient Care During Operative and Invasive Procedures*. Denver: CCI, pp. 85-129.

Module 2: Review of preoperative medications — Pages 41-43

Case Study Activity — Matching

Match Mrs. M's current medications to their action:

Glucophage: **C**

A. diuretic; inhibits sodium reabsorption

Hydrochlorothiazide: **A**

B. Nonsteroidal anti-inflammatory

Gingko Biloba: **D**

C. decreases hepatic glucose production, increases insulin sensitivity

Naproxen: **B**

D. memory enhancer (controversial)

Source: epocrates online. Retrieved Jan. 31, 2013, from http://www.epocrates.com.

Case Study Activity — Critical Thinking

How does Mrs. M.'s allergy to penicillin affect the choice of prophylactic antibiotic?

Cefazolin, the drug of choice for preoperative prophylaxis as recommended by the Surgical Care Improvement Project (SCIP) initiative, should be used with caution in patients allergic to penicillin. The anesthesiologist should be consulted prior to administration of this drug.

Source: epocrates online. Retrieved Jan. 31, 2013, from http://www.epocrates.com.

Which of Mrs. M.'s medications could influence the surgical procedure? Why?

Mrs. M. is taking both a nonsteroidal anti-inflammatory and gingko biloba. Taken together, these two drugs increase the risk for bleeding.

Source: Rothrock, J. (2011). *Alexander's Care of the Patient in Surgery.* (14th ed.). St. Louis: Mosby, p. 1252.

Mrs. M.'s diuretic puts her at risk for electrolyte imbalance, specifically potassium. Potassium regulates skeletal and cardiac muscle contraction and nerve impulses.

Source: Rothrock, J. (2011). *Alexander's Care of the Patient in Surgery.* (14th ed.). St. Louis: Mosby, p. 44.

Mrs. M. has been NPO, yet took her Glucophage this am, putting her at risk for hypoglycemia.

Source: epocrates online. Retrieved April 19, 2013, from http://www.epocrates.com.

Module 3: Initiation of the Universal Protocol — Pages 43-45

Activity — Fill in the Blank

Preoperative verification to prevent ***wrong patient, site,*** or ***procedure*** includes ensuring that all relevant documents are available prior to the procedure.

What documents can be used to verify the patient's procedure?

The history and physical, surgical consent, laboratory values, blood transfusion consent, anesthesia consent, imaging studies.

> Source: Phippen, et al. (2009). *Competency for Safe Patient Care During Operative and Invasive Procedures*. Denver: CCI, pp. 140-143.

What components of the Universal Protocol need to be incorporated in the preoperative area?

1. Verification of patient using two identifiers
2. Marking the operative site

> Source: Rothrock, J. (2011). *Alexander's Care of the Patient in Surgery*. (14th ed.). St. Louis: Mosby, p. 19.

Activity — Critical Thinking

For the following "never events," identify the corresponding AORN standard, recommended practice, guideline, or position statement that addresses it.

1. Surgery performed on the wrong body part, the wrong patient, or the wrong procedure
   Position statement on preventing wrong-patient, wrong-site, wrong-procedure events

2. Unintended retention of a foreign object in a patient after surgery or other procedure
   Recommended practices: Prevention of retained surgical items

3. Patient death or serious disability associated with a medication error
   Recommended practices: Medication safety

4. Patient death or serious disability associated with a burn incurred from any source
   Recommended practices: Laser safety, Electrosurgery, Preoperative patient skin antisepsis

5. Hospital acquired pressure ulcer
   Recommended practices: Positioning the patient

6. Deep vein thrombosis
   Recommended practices: Prevention of deep vein thrombosis

7. Hospital acquired surgical site infections

Recommended practices: Surgical attire, Hand hygiene, Sterile technique, Traffic patterns, Environmental cleaning, Prevention of transmissible infections, Prevention of hypothermia, Preoperative patient skin antisepsis, Sterilization

Source: AORN. (2013). *Perioperative Standards and Recommended Practices*. Denver: AORN.

Activity — Mark the Site

Based on The Joint Commission guidelines, mark the illustration for a right inguinal hernia repair (open).

A line, initials, or "yes" are all acceptable, and should be drawn in right inguinal (lower right quadrant) area.

Source: Rothrock, J. (2011). *Alexander's Care of the Patient in Surgery*. (14th ed.). St. Louis: Mosby, p. 31.

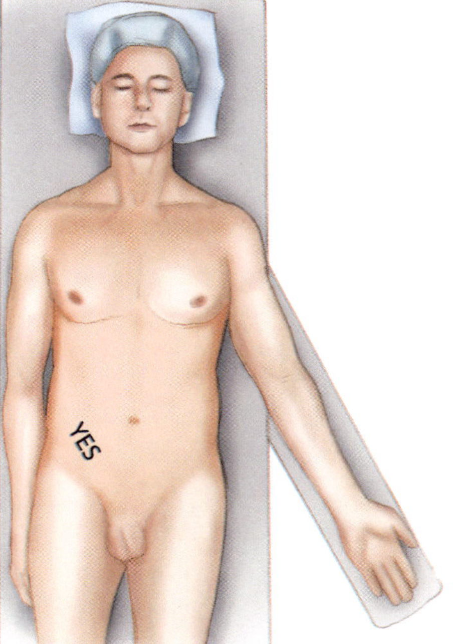

Module 4: Obtaining surgical consent — Pages 45-47

Activity — Fill in the Blank

The surgeon or practitioner performing the procedure is responsible for informing the patient about the proposed procedure in terms that he or she can understand.

It is the ***surgeon's or practitioner's*** responsibility to obtain informed consent.

Source: Rothrock, J. (2011). *Alexander's Care of the Patient in Surgery*. (14th ed.). St. Louis: Mosby, p. 45.

Activity — Critical Thinking

How does obtaining surgical consent for a child differ from that of an adult?

The person legally responsible for the child, rather than the patient, agrees to the procedure after being informed of the risks, benefits, and alternatives of the proposed procedure. Unless emancipated, a child under the age of 18 cannot sign his/her own consent. Children should be included in the discussion, and preoperative teaching should take into account age-specific needs and the extent the patient is able to understand and participate in the decision-making process. Both legal guardian and patient should have the opportunity to have questions answered.

Source: Phippen, et al. (2009). *Competency for Safe Patient Care During Operative and Invasive Procedures*. Denver: CCI, p. 1303.

Case Study Activity — Consent

Mrs. M.s' consent states that she is scheduled for a laparoscopic cholecystectomy, possible open, with cholangiograms.

1. How will you evaluate Mrs. M.'s understanding of the proposed procedure?

Ask open-ended questions to avoid leading Mrs. M. to a correct response. Have her describe in her own words the procedure and what it is for. Questions related to risks, alternatives, benefits, or other medical-related questions should be referred to the surgeon.

Source: Phippen, et al. (2009). *Competency for Safe Patient Care During Operative and Invasive Procedures*. Denver: CCI, pp. 58-59.

2. What puts Mrs. M. at risk for converting to an open procedure?

Her weight and previous abdominal surgeries

Source: Rothrock, J. (2011). *Alexander's Care of the Patient in Surgery*. (14th ed.). St. Louis: Mosby, p. 375.

Module 5: Ensuring patients' rights by providing information on advance directives, do-not-resuscitate — Pages 47-48

Activity — True or False

Under the Patient Self-Determination Act, patients have the legal right to accept or refuse medical treatment, including resuscitation, even if refusal will likely result in death.

True: Under the Patient Self-Determination Act, patients have the legal right to accept or refuse medical treatment, including resuscitation, even if refusal will likely result in death.

Source: Rothrock, J. (2011). *Alexander's Care of the Patient in Surgery*. (14th ed.). St. Louis: Mosby, p. 45.

Module 6: Pain assessment — Pages 48-50

Activity — Matching

Match the most appropriate pain rating scale to the patient identified below (answers may be used more than once)

A. 0-10 Numeric pain intensity scale

3-year-old: ***B***

B. FACES Pain rating scale

45-year-old man: ***A, C***

C. Simple descriptive pain intensity scale

23-year-old woman, does not speak English: ***B***

Source: Rothrock, J. (2011). *Alexander's Care of the Patient in Surgery.* (14th ed.). St. Louis: Mosby, p. 282.

Case Study Activity — Pain Assessment

How can you incorporate components of Mrs. M.'s age, sex, ethnicity, and culture into her pain management plan? (Note: This same format may be utilized when developing any patient's pain treatment plan.)

A good rule of thumb is to treat the patient the way she would want to be treated. A baseline pain level should be determined against which postoperative pain can then be measured. Chronic pain should be considered in the pain management plan.

Mrs. M.'s previous experiences with surgical pain and what was effective in alleviating it should be included in the plan of care. A self-report tool should be agreed upon and communicated to other health care workers. Mrs. M. should determine the acceptable level of pain, and interventions should be directed toward reaching that level.

Preoperative teaching will help Mrs. M. understand what type of pain to expect, what will be done to treat it (both pharmacologic and nonpharmacologic interventions) and her role in participating in pain management. Her family should be included in this discussion as appropriate.

Source: Rothrock, J. (2011). *Alexander's Care of the Patient in Surgery.* (14th ed.). St. Louis: Mosby, pp. 280-287.

Module 7: Development of nursing diagnoses — Pages 50-52

Activity — Matching

Match the term to its correct definition:

Etiology: **B**

Nursing diagnosis: **F**

Nursing intervention: **D**

Problem: **E**

Sign: **A**

Symptom: **C**

A. Objective information obtained through the five senses

B. Cause of a disease supported by medical data

C. Subjective information obtained through what the patient tells you

D. Actions for which the perioperative nurse is accountable

E. Any condition that requires a nursing intervention

F. Identification of a real or potential patient problem or risk

Source: Venes, D. (ed.). (2009). *Tabor's Cyclopedic Medical Dictionary.* Philadelphia, PA: F.A. Davis Co.

Case Study Activity — Nursing Diagnoses

From your interpretation of Mrs. M.'s assessment data, formulate nursing diagnoses to address each identified problem or potential problem. Write your nursing diagnoses in the boxes next to your "major problem" in your concept map on the CD. Not all of your "major problems" may have a corresponding nursing diagnosis. ***Sample answers added to the map below.***

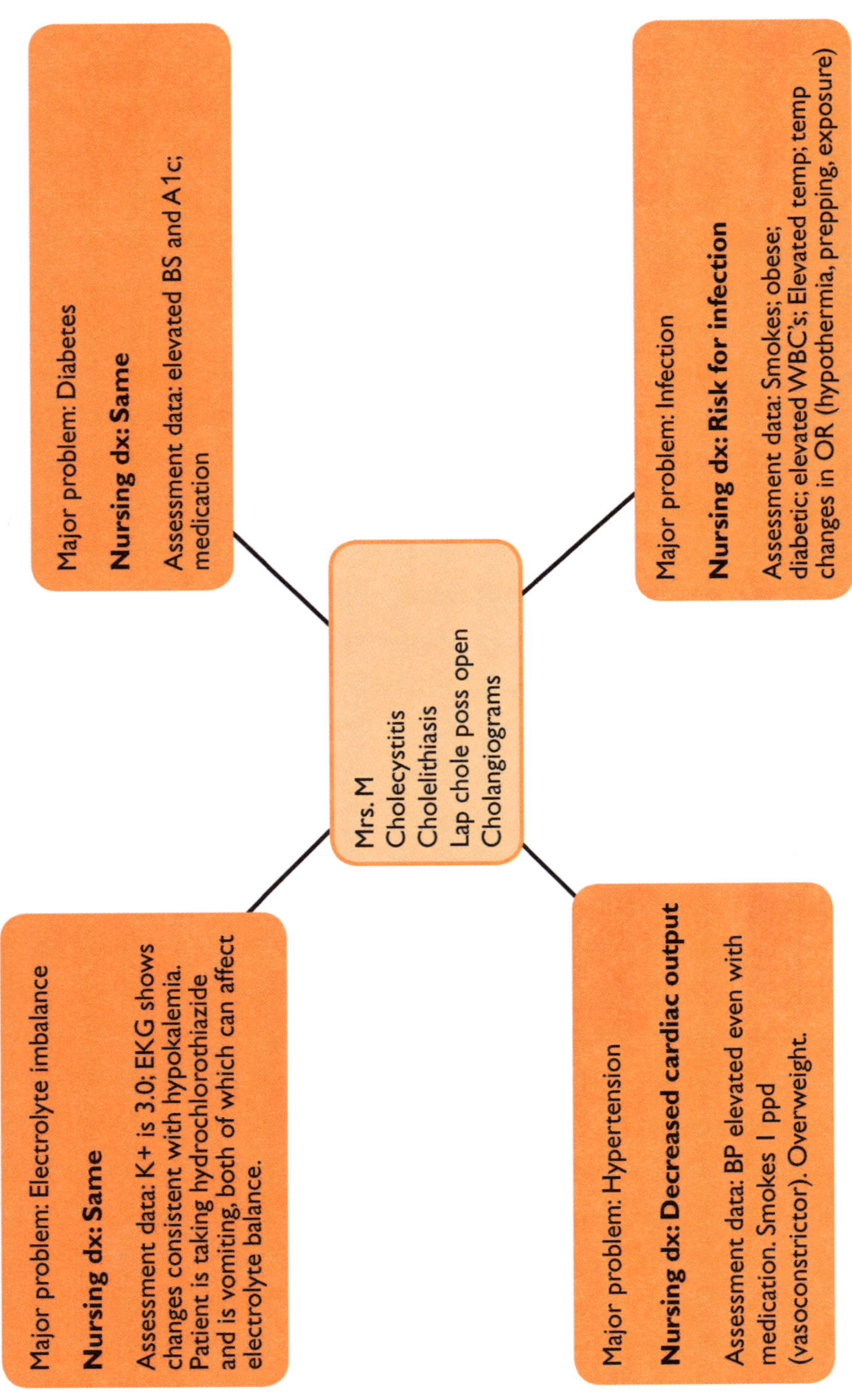

CHAPTER 2:
Identify Expected Outcomes and Develop an Individualized Plan of Care

Introduction

Perioperative nurses perform the important functions of setting priorities and identifying desirable outcomes during the planning phase of the nursing process.

The plan of care is derived from nursing diagnoses and is developed through effective communication with the patient and other parties as appropriate. The plan should be patient centered, be culturally considerate, and provide for continuity of care. After all, the intraoperative experience is just one event in the patient's life. Encouraging the patient to take an active role in the overall plan preserves his or her autonomy, privacy, dignity, and rights.

Organizing the components of patient care can be confusing, so different methods have been developed to categorize and define nursing terminology and actions. The *Perioperative Nursing Data Set* (PNDS) is a standardized language that has incorporated perioperative nursing diagnoses, interventions, and outcomes (AORN, 2011). The PNDS will be used throughout this chapter as the template for the development of care plans. It is not the only taxonomy used in the nursing profession, but it is specific to the perioperative arena. Many electronic medical records have incorporated the PNDS into their charting systems. The glossary in this chapter includes definitions for the terms used in the PNDS, and frequently used nursing diagnoses are provided in Chapter 1 on page 51.

This chapter provides opportunities to identify expected outcomes and develop plans of care for the surgical patient based on your assessment. Measurable patient data are used to develop specific outcomes. Suggestions for individualizing the plan of care are provided. For the purposes of this chapter, we will continue to build on the information captured in the concept map on the CD begun in Chapter 1 (page 39).

Module 1: Develop Measurable Patient Outcomes from Patient Assessment Data and Nursing Diagnoses

Outcomes can be considered the goals or desired end results of nursing, or "nurse sensitive" interventions. In the case of perioperative nursing, they are what we want our patients to be able to do or exhibit at the end of a procedure. By developing expected outcomes, the perioperative nurse is able to:

1. Select appropriate nursing interventions to be used in the plan of care.
2. Determine a baseline against which to measure success of the intervention.
3. Identify reasonable time frames in which to achieve goals.

Outcomes should be realistic, relevant to the patient's condition, based on available resources, and written in measurable terms. Interdisciplinary collaboration and patient expectations are equally important in helping to identify the best outcomes for the patient.

Competency Outcomes

To successfully complete the activities in this module, you will need to be able to:

1. Construct perioperative patient outcome statements based on assessment data and nursing diagnoses.
2. List three advantages of developing patient outcomes that can be included in a plan of care.

Recommended Readings

Alexander's Care of the Patient in Surgery. (2011, 14th ed.), Chapter 1: Concepts basic to perioperative nursing; Unit II: Surgical interventions.

AORN. (2013). *Perioperative Standards and Recommended Practices,* Section II: Recommended practices for perioperative nursing; Section III: Guidance statements.

Berry and Kohn's Operating Room Technique. (2013, 12th ed.), Chapter 2: Foundations of perioperative patient care standards.

Competency for Safe Patient Care During Operative and Invasive Procedures. (2009). Chapter 1: Systems-in-contingency: A conceptual model; Chapter 5: Preparation of the patient for the procedure.

Key Words

Measurable, nursing intervention, nurse sensitive, outcome, PNDS

Activity — Short Answer

Three benefits of identifying expected outcomes are that the perioperative nurse will be able to:

1. *Select appropriate interventions*
2. *Determine a baseline*
3. *Determine realistic time frames to achieve goals*

> ### "Go To" Case Study Activity
>
> For the concept map you have developed on the CD for Mrs. M., add patient outcomes to the appropriate boxes.

Module 2: Develop an Individualized Plan of Care

Plans of care are developed using the information obtained during the patient assessment and corresponding nursing diagnoses. The perioperative registered nurse must prioritize patient problems, work within a multidisciplinary environment, develop criteria for evaluation, and utilize evidence-based practice — in the five minutes taken to interview and assess the patient! The plan shapes the course of care for the patient, and for that reason, it should be based on the most current best practices. It should be easily understood and accessed by all health care providers; therefore, clear, comprehensive documentation of nursing interventions is needed to validate nursing practice and patient outcomes.

Caring for patients across the lifespan requires that the perioperative nurse applies the nursing process to meet the age-specific needs of the patient. Various theories address psychosocial, sensory, and aging-associated phases of human growth and development (Rothrock, 2011). Regardless of a patient's age, the perioperative nurse develops a care plan that is directed toward avoiding or resolving patient problems.

Competency Outcomes

To successfully complete the activities in this module, you will need to be able to:

1. Develop a plan of care specific to the patient based on age, developmental level, and nursing diagnoses.
2. Collaborate with the interdisciplinary health care team in addressing identified patient needs.

Recommended Readings

Alexander's Care of the Patient in Surgery. (2011, 14th ed.), Chapter 1: Concepts basic to perioperative nursing; Unit II: Surgical interventions.

Perioperative Standards and Recommended Practices. (2013), Section 1: Standards of perioperative nursing; Section II: Recommended practices for perioperative nursing; Section III: Guidance statements.

Berry and Kohn's Operating Room Technique. (2013, 12th ed.), Chapter 2: Foundations of perioperative patient care standards; Chapter 7: The patient: The reason for your existence; Chapter 9: Perioperative geriatrics; Chapter 11: Ambulatory surgery centers and alternative surgical locations; Chapter 21: Preoperative preparation of the patient.

Competency for Safe Patient Care During Operative and Invasive Procedures. (2009). Chapter 2: Competency assessment; Chapter 5: Preparation of the patient for the procedure.

Key Words

Age-specific, nursing diagnosis, nursing interventions, nursing process, patient problems, plan of care

Activity — Fill in the Blank

Fill in the patient outcome and nursing interventions for each of the following scenarios:

1. Nursing diagnosis: Knowledge deficit related to procedure
    Assessment data:
    Objective: Patient is scheduled for laparoscopic bilateral tubal ligation.
    Subjective: Patient states: "I'll be so happy when I don't have such terrible cramps with my periods anymore. Maybe this means I'll be able to get pregnant now."

    Patient outcome: ____

    Nursing interventions: ____

2. Nursing diagnosis: Risk for infection
    Assessment data:
    Objective: Patient is scheduled for ventral hernia repair with mesh. She is on long-term corticosteroids for the treatment of systemic lupus erythrematosis (SLE). Assessment of skin integrity shows multiple areas of bruising on arms and legs.

Subjective: "My skin is like tissue paper, and I take forever to heal, even when it's just a small cut or scrape."

Patient outcome: ____

Nursing interventions: ____

3. Nursing diagnosis: Risk for developing hypothermia
   Assessment data:
   Objective: 3-month-old boy scheduled for cleft lip repair. Patient's temperature (temporal artery) is 37.2° C.

   Patient outcome: ____

   Nursing interventions: ____

4. Nursing diagnosis: Risk for perioperative positioning injury
   Assessment data:
   Objective: Patient is scheduled for transurethral resection of the prostate (TURP). Subjective: "I feel like the bionic man. I've had both hips replaced."

   Patient outcome: ____

   Nursing interventions: ____

Additional Readings/Resources

Doerflinger, D.M.C. (2009). Older adult surgical patients: Presentation and challenges. *AORN Journal, 90*(2), 223-242. Bonus: Examination questions follow the article.

> ### "Go To" Case Study Activity
>
> For each box in your concept map on the CD, list the nursing interventions needed to meet the identified outcomes/goals.

Module 3: Incorporate Patient Education Into the Plan of Care

Teaching is an essential role of the professional nurse. Assessing the patient's readiness to learn, identifying barriers to learning, and establishing prior knowledge of the event provide a preliminary framework from which the nurse establishes a teaching-learning plan specific to the patient's needs. The perioperative nurse acts as the patient advocate and practices according to the *ANA Code of Ethics for Nurses* (AORN, 2013).

As individuals, patients experience a range of responses to the surgical experience. Many variables affect an individual's ability to learn — the type of surgery, reason for surgery, available resources and support services, age of the patient, and cultural and spiritual needs. Surgery is a stressful event, and it affects the patient's ability to hear and process information.

Facilities must comply with The Joint Commission regulations on patient education in order to be accredited, but teaching our patients goes beyond legal requirements. Patients who understand their treatment plan are less likely to be readmitted or have infections or other complications. A knowledgeable patient is one of the most cost-effective goals a facility can strive to achieve.

The immediate preoperative setting, however, is not an ideal environment for patient education. Anxiety, time constraints, and preoperative medications do not provide an atmosphere conducive to learning new materials or retaining information.

The perioperative nurse is wise to prioritize and limit teaching strategies to:

1. What does the patient already know?
2. What does the patient need to know?
3. What factors will enhance or inhibit the learning experience?
4. What is the best method for sharing information?
5. How will I know that the patient understands what has been taught?

Competency Outcomes

To successfully complete the activities in this module, you will need to be able to:

1. Incorporate patient rights and responsibilities into a teaching plan.
2. Recognize the impact of surgical stressors (medications, pain, and anxiety) on the ability to learn.
3. Identify community and institutional resources based on identified patient needs.
4. Incorporate The Joint Commission's requirements for patient education into a teaching plan.
5. Identify barriers and aids to learning.

Recommended Readings

Alexander's Care of the Patient in Surgery. (2011, 14th ed.), Unit II: Surgical interventions; Unit III: Special considerations.

Perioperative Standards and Recommended Practices. (2013), Exhibit B: Perioperative explications for the ANA Code of Ethics for Nurses, pp. 21-42.

Berry and Kohn's Operating Room Technique. (2013, 12th ed.), Chapter 2: Foundations of perioperative patient care standards; Chapter 21: Preoperative preparation of the patient.

Competency for Safe Patient Care During Operative and Invasive Procedures. (2009). Chapter 5: Preparation of the patient for the procedure; Chapter 18: Facilitate care after the procedure.

Key Words

Age-specific, barriers, patient education

Case Study Activity

1. How can you determine what Mrs. M. already knows about her upcoming surgery?

2. What does Mrs. M. need to know to participate in her plan of care?

3. What are Mrs. M.'s strengths/barriers to learning?

4. How can you determine that Mrs. M. understands what you have told her?

5. What resources can you recommend to assist Mrs. M. postoperatively with the problems you've identified? How will she access these resources?

Additional Readings/Resources:

Kruzik, N. (2009). Benefits of preoperative education for adult elective surgery patients. *AORN Journal, 90*(3), 381-387.

Ortoleva, C. (2010). An approach to consistent patient education. *AORN Journal, 92*(4), 437-444.

Sorenson, H.L., Card, C.A., Malley, M.T., & Strzelecki, J. M. (2009). Using a collaborative child life approach for continuous surgical preparation. *AORN Journal, 90*(4), 557-566.

Chapter Summary

Managing the care of perioperative patients requires critical thinking, independent judgment in clinical decision making, collaboration among all other health care professionals, and an ethical code to guide practice. By using the nursing process, the perioperative nurse prioritizes patient problems identified by objective and subjective data.

Patient centered outcomes are determined from the nursing diagnoses and are written in measurable terms. Nursing interventions are designed to achieve the established outcomes, and through evaluation, the outcomes may be renegotiated and revised.

The examples found throughout this chapter reflect perioperative patient outcomes, outcome definitions, and outcome indicators. Note that the indicators are observable and measurable. The goal for the development of a plan of care is to identify and address the needs of the patient through the provision of quality, evidence-based practice.

Glossary

Family — For purposes of this guide, significant others and extended family are included in the term "family."

Health care team — The providers of patient care services who are required to provide direct patient care to help the patient achieve a positive outcome. Support services include but are not limited to pharmacy, radiology, blood bank, housekeeping, etc.

North American Nursing Diagnosis Association (NANDA) — The group that has developed a list of 155 accepted nursing diagnoses to ensure that documentation in all areas of nursing use consistent, comparable terminology. (www.nanda.org) Also see *Perioperative Nursing Data Set.*

Nursing diagnosis — A statement derived from the nursing assessment data that provides the framework for nursing interventions that enable the patient to attain specific desired outcomes. It is structured using standardized nursing nomenclature. Also see North American Nursing Diagnosis Association and *Perioperative Nursing Data Set.*

Nursing process — The critical thinking a nurse uses to assess the health status of patients, identify problems, develop and implement plans of care, and evaluate the patients' responses to that care.

Perioperative Nursing Data Set (PNDS) — The perioperative nursing vocabulary guidebook that provides nursing diagnosis, nursing interventions, and patient outcomes statements specific to the perioperative environment.

Terms specific to the PNDS:

Domain — The four overall divisions of the conceptual framework of the *Perioperative Nursing Data Set.* All interventions and expected outcomes relate to one or more domains. The four domains are Safety, Physiologic Responses, Behavioral Responses, and the Health System.

Outcome — Outcomes are designed to direct and evaluate patient care and are part of the overall plan of care. The perioperative nurse in collaboration with the patient formulates the outcomes from the nursing diagnoses. In the case of the PNDS, the outcomes serve as positive statements reflecting expected achievement of identified goals (AORN, 2011). Outcomes should be written in a concise, measurable, and realistic manner. Documentation of the plan of care, expected outcomes, and nursing interventions provides a means for evaluation.

Outcome indicator — Measures of performance that link nursing interventions to outcomes. Typically, an indicator is a clinical finding, although it may be an administrative quality benchmark (as in documentation) or a fiscal value (as in cost-effective measures).

Applicable nursing diagnosis — A statement derived from the nursing assessment data that provides the framework for nursing interventions. The diagnosis may be a real or potential problem. It is structured using standardized nursing terms.

Intervention — An action taken based on patient assessment data with the intention of achieving one or more expected patient outcomes.

Evaluation — The final step in the nursing process in which success of interventions in meeting outcomes is measured.

Plan of care (or care plan) — A result of a systematic process of identifying expected patient outcomes and determining how to achieve them. It includes the list of interventions necessary to reach the expected outcome. The plan of care directs all nursing care activities related to each patient.

Support services — Pharmacy, radiology, blood bank, laboratories, environmental services (i.e., housekeeping), biomedical engineering, etc.

Transfer — Moving a patient from one place to another (e.g., to or from a bed or stretcher).

Transport — Moving a patient via a device (e.g., wheelchair, stretcher, wagon).

References

AORN. (2011). *Perioperative Nursing Data Set* (3rd ed.). Denver: AORN, Inc.

AORN. (2013). Exhibit B: Perioperative explications for the ANA Code of Ethics for nurses. In *Perioperative Standards and Recommended Practices*. Denver: AORN, Inc.

Phillips, N. (2013). *Berry and Kohn's Operating Room Technique* (12th ed.). St. Louis: Mosby.

Phippen, M.L., Ulmer, B.C., & Wells, M. P. (2009). *Competency for Safe Patient Care During Operative and Invasive Procedures.* Denver: CCI.

Rothrock, J.C. (Ed.). (2011). *Alexander's Care of the Patient in Surgery* (14th ed.). St. Louis: Mosby.

Answers to Chapter 2 Activities

Module 1: Develop measurable patient outcomes from patient assessment data and nursing diagnoses — Pages 68-69

Activity — Short Answer

Three benefits of identifying expected outcomes are that the perioperative nurse will be able to:
1. *Select appropriate nursing interventions to be used in the plan of care.*
2. *Determine a baseline against which to measure success of the intervention.*
3. *Identify realistic time frames in which to achieve goals.*

Sources: Phillips, N. (2013). *Berry and Kohn Operating Room Technique* (12th ed.). St. Louis: Mosby Elsevier, pp. 32-33. Rothrock, J. (2011). *Alexander's Care of the Patient in Surgery* (14th ed.). St. Louis: Mosby, pp. 7-8.

"Go To" Case Study Activity

From the concept map you have developed on the CD for Mrs. M., add patient outcomes to the appropriate boxes. *Examples are provided on the next page, but are not to be considered all-inclusive.*

Sources: Rothrock, J. (2011). *Alexander's Care of the Patient in Surgery* (14th ed.). St. Louis: Mosby, pp. 7-11. AORN. (2013). *Perioperative Standards and Recommended Practices,* Sections II and III. Denver: AORN.

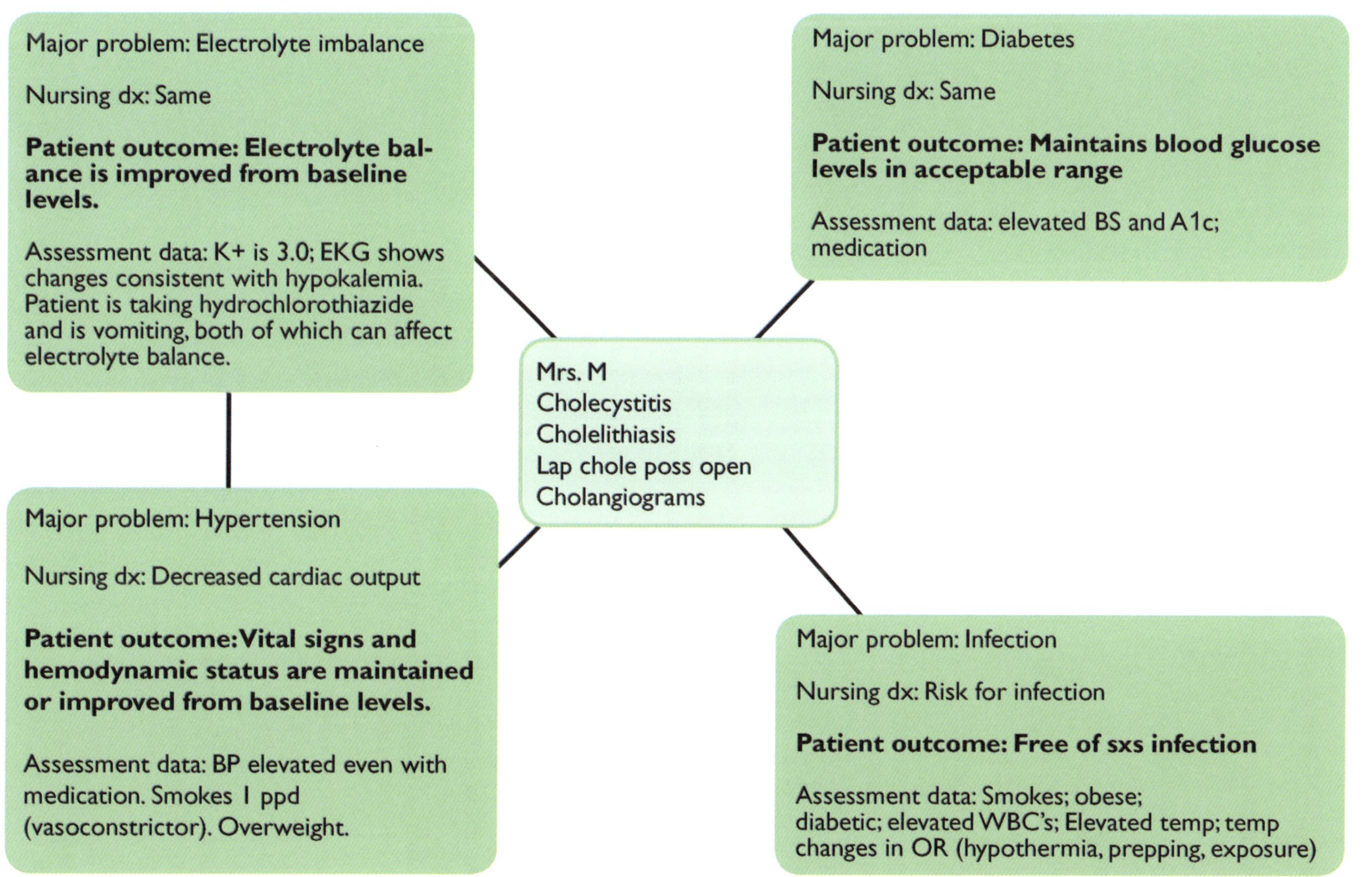
Major problem: Electrolyte imbalance

Nursing dx: Same

Patient outcome: Electrolyte balance is improved from baseline levels.

Assessment data: K+ is 3.0; EKG shows changes consistent with hypokalemia. Patient is taking hydrochlorothiazide and is vomiting, both of which can affect electrolyte balance.

Major problem: Diabetes

Nursing dx: Same

Patient outcome: Maintains blood glucose levels in acceptable range

Assessment data: elevated BS and A1c; medication

Mrs. M
Cholecystitis
Cholelithiasis
Lap chole poss open
Cholangiograms

Major problem: Hypertension

Nursing dx: Decreased cardiac output

Patient outcome: Vital signs and hemodynamic status are maintained or improved from baseline levels.

Assessment data: BP elevated even with medication. Smokes 1 ppd (vasoconstrictor). Overweight.

Major problem: Infection

Nursing dx: Risk for infection

Patient outcome: Free of sxs infection

Assessment data: Smokes; obese; diabetic; elevated WBC's; Elevated temp; temp changes in OR (hypothermia, prepping, exposure)

Module 2: Develop an individualized plan of care — Pages 69-71

Activity — Fill in the Blank

Fill in the patient outcome and nursing interventions for each of the following scenarios. *Examples are provided below, but are not to be considered all-inclusive.*

1. Nursing diagnosis: Knowledge deficit related to procedure
    Assessment data:
    Objective: Patient is scheduled for laparoscopic bilateral tubal ligation.
    Subjective: Patient states: "I'll be so happy when I don't have such terrible cramps with my periods anymore. Maybe this means I'll be able to get pregnant now."

    Patient outcome: Patient demonstrates knowledge of physiologic responses to surgical procedure.
    Nursing interventions: Implement the Universal Protocol (correct patient, correct surgery, correct site). Confirm stated procedure with schedule and consent. Notify surgeon of discrepancy between patient's understanding of procedure and scheduled surgery.

2. Nursing diagnosis: Risk for infection
    Assessment data:
    Objective: Patient is scheduled for ventral hernia repair with mesh. She is on long-term corticosteroids for the treatment of systemic lupus erythrematosis (SLE). Assessment of skin integrity shows multiple areas of bruising on arms and legs.
    Subjective: "My skin is like tissue paper, and I take forever to heal, even when it's just a small cut or scrape."

    Patient outcome: The patient is free of signs and symptoms of infection.
    Nursing interventions: Implement and maintain aseptic technique; implement protective measures to prevent injury to skin.

3. Nursing diagnosis: Risk for developing hypothermia
    Assessment data:
    Objective: 3-month-old boy scheduled for cleft lip repair. Patient's temperature (temporal artery) is 37.2° C.

    Patient outcome: Patient is at or returning to normothermia at conclusion of procedure.
    Nursing interventions: Limit skin exposure to operative site; implement thermoregulation measures (prewarming, warming devices, warm IV fluids, increase room temperature, provide equipment for anesthesia provider to humidify/warm anesthetic gases). Use a reliable site for measuring core temperature.

4. Nursing diagnosis: Risk for perioperative positioning injury
    Assessment data:
    Objective: Patient is scheduled for transurethral resection of the prostate (TURP).
    Subjective: "I feel like the bionic man. I've had both hips replaced."

Patient outcome: Patient is free of signs and symptoms of injury related to positioning; regains normal mobility postoperatively.
Nursing interventions: Obtain positioning aids and padding. Avoid hyperabduction of hips/ leaning on inner thighs. Avoid high stirrups and use boot stirrups if possible. Position stirrups at the same height and ensure that devices are securely attached to OR bed. Limit time in lithotomy position by efficient use of OR time and resources. Legs should be lifted and removed from stirrups slowly and simultaneously; return legs to bed one at a time if possible. Evaluate for signs and symptoms of injury related to positioning.

Sources: AORN. (2013). Recommended practices: Sterile technique; Positioning the patient in the perioperative practice setting; Prevention of hypothermia. In *Perioperative Standards and Recommended Practices.* Denver: AORN, Inc. Rothrock, J.C. (Ed.). (2011). *Alexander's Care of the Patient in Surgery* (14th ed.). St. Louis: Mosby, pp. 7-12.

"Go To" Case Study Activity

For each box in your concept map on the CD, list the nursing interventions needed to meet the identified outcomes/goals. ***Examples are provided on the following page, but are not to be considered all-inclusive.***

Module 3: Incorporate patient education into the plan of care — Pages 71-74

Case Study Activity

1. How can you determine what Mrs. M. already knows about her upcoming surgery?

Ask Mrs. M. to describe in her own words her planned surgery, the reason(s) for it, and the proposed plan of care (length of stay, type of anesthesia, etc.).

2. What does Mrs. M. need to know to participate in her plan of care?

Mrs. M. needs to be provided information on the perioperative plan of care in terms that she understands. Adequate time needs to be provided to answer her and her family's questions. Information needs to be prioritized so that the most important information (surgery and immediate postoperative period) are covered.

3. What are Mrs. M.'s strengths/barriers to learning?

Strengths:
 Strong family support system
 Familiar with health care environment through employment setting
 Cultural definitions of health and wellness

Barriers:

Stressful environment	***Anxiety/fear***
Medications	***Cultural definitions of health and wellness***

(continued on page 81)

"Go To" Case Study Activity

SAMPLE Concept map listing the nursing interventions needed to meet the identified outcomes/goals.

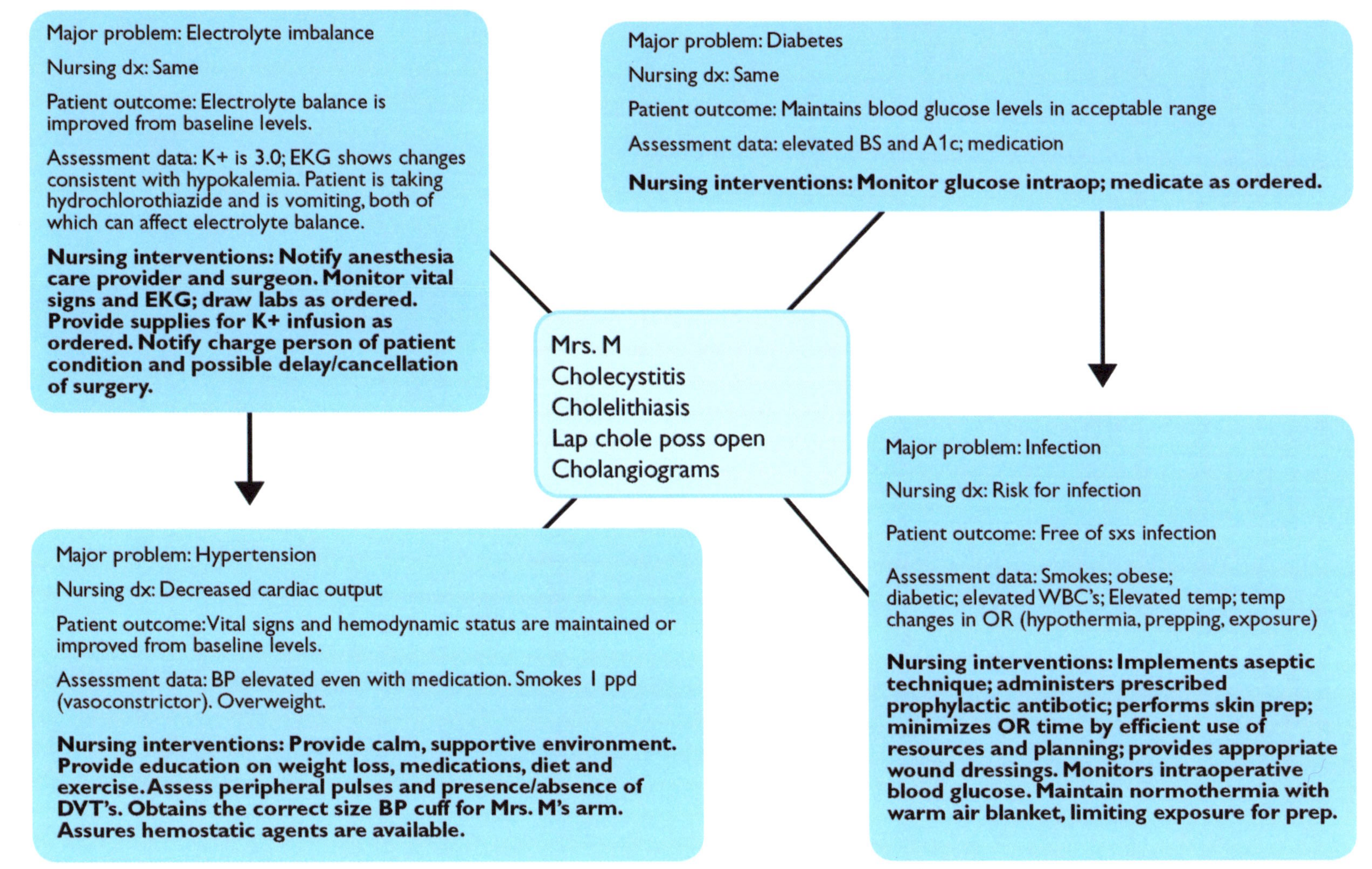

4. How can you determine that Mrs. M. understands what you have told her?

By having her teach back or demonstrate back (as appropriate) the information she has received.

Source: Phippen et al. (2009). *Competency for Safe Patient Care During Operative and Invasive Procedures*. Denver: CCI, pp. 572-577.

5. What resources can you recommend to assist Mrs. M. postoperatively with the problems you've identified? How will she access these resources?

** Note: the following references are examples only; CCI does not endorse any of these programs or organizations. Web site addresses were accurate as of Jan. 31, 2013.*

Hospital-based wellness classes: Check with your facility's case manager for a list of resources that are available both in-house and in the community.

Smoking cessation resources:
- ***American Heart Association: Smoking effects.*** ***http://www.heart.org/HEARTORG/search/searchResults.jsp?_dyncharset=ISO-8859-1&q=smoking+effects***
- ***Smokefree.gov: http://smokefree.gov/***
- ***Centers for Disease Control and Prevention (CDC): Smoking and tobacco use: Quit smoking.*** ***http://www.cdc.gov/tobacco/quit_smoking/index.htm***

Weight control information: Multiple programs are available. Mrs. M. needs to consult with her family physician to develop a plan that incorporates sensible exercise and nutrition.

Diabetic education: American Diabetes Association (www.diabetes.org/)

Malignant hyperthermia information: MHAUS (www.mhaus.org/)

Latex allergy information: Medline plus (www.nlm.nih.gov/medlineplus/latexallergy.html)

NOTES

CHAPTER 3:
Intraoperative Activities

Introduction

The intraoperative phase begins when the patient enters the operating room (OR) or procedure area and ends when the patient is transferred to the postanesthesia care unit (PACU), intensive care unit (ICU), or other level of care. During this phase, the patient receives anesthetic agents; is positioned, prepped, and draped; and undergoes the operative or invasive procedure. The practice of perioperative nursing requires a combination of active assessment, collaboration, technical skills, and critical thinking skills unique to this area of nursing.

As one member of a multidisciplinary team who focuses solely on the surgical patient's needs, the perioperative RN serves as the primary patient advocate while coordinating the efforts of all team members toward the goal of optimal patient outcomes. This already Herculean task is compounded by today's ever-expanding arsenal of new technology including robotics, remote surgeries, novel applications of minimally invasive procedures, and "biologic" implant and graft materials. Our patients are sicker, our time spent with them is shorter, and both the consumer and the facility demand quality, efficient, cost-effective health care experiences. Today's perioperative RN is challenged to continually update an existing knowledge base through lifelong learning and ongoing education.

This chapter will help you review the competencies needed to safely care for the patient in the intraoperative phase of surgery. The plan of care developed for our patient in Chapters 1 and 2 will be incorporated into intraoperative nursing interventions. Concepts including maintenance of aseptic technique, risk factors for environmental injury, emotional and sociocultural issues, and health system and regulatory standards, regulation, and guidelines are applied to clinical learning activities.

Module 1: Introduction of the Patient to the Operative/Procedure Area

Every patient has unique physical and behavioral responses to stresses encountered during the surgical procedure, regardless of the setting. These responses must be taken into account as the perioperative nurse incorporates appropriate nursing interventions and evaluates their effectiveness. The first task when the patient enters the operative or procedure area is to provide a safe environment that is supportive of not only a patient's physiologic needs, but also his/her beliefs, personal rights, and dignity.

Competency Outcomes

To successfully complete the activities in this module, you will need to be able to:

1. Appraise behavioral responses of the patient and family to the surgical experience.
2. Review components of the time-out.
3. Design activities to address common physiologic responses to the surgical experience.
4. Apply measures to promote patient comfort and safety.

Recommended Readings

Alexander's Care of the Patient in Surgery. (2011, 14th ed.), Chapter 2: Patient safety and risk management; Chapter 3: Infection prevention and control in the perioperative setting; Chapter 5: Positioning the patient for surgery.

Perioperative Standards and Recommended Practices. (2013), Recommended practices:
- Prevention of unplanned hypothermia.
- Transfer of patient care information.
- Prevention of deep vein thrombosis.

Perioperative Standards and Recommended Practices. (2013), Guidance statement:
- Safe patient handling and movement.

Berry and Kohn's Operating Room Technique. (2013, 12th ed.), Chapter 2: Foundations of perioperative patient care standards; Chapter 7: The patient: The reason for your existence; Chapter 11: Ambulatory surgery centers and alternative surgical locations; Chapter 21: Preoperative preparation of the patient; Chapter 25: Coordinated roles of the scrub person and the circulating nurse.

Competency for Safe Patient Care During Operative and Invasive Procedures. (2009), Chapter 4: Legal, regulatory, and ethical considerations; Chapter 6: Transfer the patient; Chapter 7: Assist the anesthesia provider; Chapter 11: Provide instruments, equipment, and supplies; Chapter 13: Physiologicly monitor the patient.

Key Words

Behavioral response, beliefs, confidentiality, culture, hypothermia, intraoperative, knowledge deficit, patient coping mechanisms, patient education, patient privacy, patient transfer, physiologic response, spirituality, stress, time-out, venous stasis

Activity — Short Answer

Who is included in a time-out prior to surgery?

Everyone involved in procedure
Surgeon, anesthesia, circ, scrub, rep

Case Study Activity

What risk factors does Mrs. M. have for developing a deep vein thrombosis?

obesity, smoking, positioning (reverse Trend.)

Activity — Critical Thinking

Your patient, scheduled for a total hip arthroplasty, has stated that her religious beliefs prevent her from accepting a blood transfusion. What are your choices in fluid management that will respect her wishes?

Volume expanders
Dextran - large molecules (colloid)   Autotransfusion
Saline / Ringers (crystalloid)
Heta starch + Penta starch
Hespan (colloid)
Albumin (colloid)

Case Study Activity

1. When should Mrs. M.'s preoperative antibiotic be administered? When should it be discontinued?   *w/in 60 mins of incision.*
D 24°

2. What should be included in Mrs. M.'s time-out?

Sx site per consent
allergies
DOB
ID
ABT
implants
& blood

Continued on next page.

Case Study Activity *(continued)*

3. Mrs. M. wonders "what all the fuss is about" concerning keeping her warm. She states, "In 5 minutes, I'll be asleep, and won't even know if I'm cold or not." What do you tell her?

SE of hypothermia

↑ risk infection

abn ⊘ rhythms → VT

↑ risk of bleeding (inhibits plt aggregation)

alters metabolism (Δ bodies reaction to meds)

4. From your preoperative assessment you learned that Mrs. M.'s maternal grandmother died during surgery to remove her gallbladder in 1954. Mrs. M. states "I'm really worried that the same thing is going to happen to me." How would you address Mrs. M.'s concern? What nursing interventions can you employ to decrease her anxiety?

Offer comfort + support. Find out if anyone else has had any trouble. Alert anesthesia about poss of MH.

5. Physiologic responses to the stress of the surgical procedure and Mrs. M.'s health assessment can trigger some unique situations for the management of her care. In reviewing her preoperative assessment, what physiologic responses might you as her intraoperative nurse encounter?

<table>
<tr><td>

"Go To" Activity — Check It Out!

Go to Question #18, Age-specific care; Question #20, Pediatrics; and Question #42, Alternatives to blood transfusion, under the Perioperative question of the week tab on your CD for additional critical-thinking activities.

</td><td>

"Go To" Activity — Skill Building

Review your facility's policies and procedures on prevention of deep vein thrombosis and hypothermia and compare them to AORN's standards and recommended practices.

Identify the resources in your facility that can be used to address your patient's spiritual needs.

</td></tr>
</table>

Additional Reading/Resources

Bailey, L. (2010). Strategies for decreasing patient anxiety in the perioperative setting. *AORN Journal*, *92*(4), 445-460.

Burlingame, B.L. (2007). Deep vein thrombosis. *AORN Journal*, *85*(1), 189-192.

Griffin, A.T., & Yancey, V. (2009). Spiritual dimensions of the perioperative experience. *AORN Journal*, *89*(5), 875-882.

Hegarty, J., Walsh, I., Burton, A., Murphy, S., et al. (2009). Nurses' knowledge of inadvertent hypothermia. *AORN Journal*, *89*(4), 701-713.

Norton, E.K., & Rangel, S.J. (2010). Implementing a pediatric surgical safety checklist in the OR and beyond. *AORN Journal*, *92*(1), 61-71.

Waters, T., Baptiste, A., Short, M., Plante-Mallon L., et al. (2011). AORN ergonomic tool 1: Lateral transfer of a patient from a stretcher to an OR bed. *AORN Journal*, *93*(3). 334-339.

Weirich, T.L. (2008). Hypothermia/warming protocols: Why are they not widely used in the OR? *AORN Journal*, *87*(2), 333-344.

Module 2: Support Safe Practices Regarding Anesthesia Provider, Surgeon, and Nurse Administered Medications

Although the number of drugs actually administered by the perioperative nurse may be quite small, the nurse is still responsible for their safe delivery to the sterile field. The responsibility for choosing the right drug in the right dose for the right patient, given via the right route, at the right time, for the right reason, and with the right documentation, is shared by all members of the surgical team. The perioperative nurse's role and responsibility related to anesthetic management of the intraoperative patient varies in scope, depending upon the presence of an anesthesia care provider, the health status of the patient, and the anesthetic technique employed. As nursing scope of practice expands to administering and monitoring drugs traditionally given by an anesthesia care provider, the perioperative nurse acquires additional skills in assessing and managing the patient undergoing moderate sedation.

Competency Outcomes

To successfully complete the activities in this module, you will need to be able to:

1. Differentiate nursing actions utilized in assisting the anesthesia care provider with regional and general anesthesia.
2. Identify key points in providing safe care for the anesthetized patient.
3. Examine the role of the nurse in monitoring a patient undergoing moderate sedation.
4. Review pharmacology of drugs administered during the intraoperative phase.

Recommended Readings

Alexander's Care of the Patient in Surgery. (2011, 14th ed.), Chapter 2: Patient safety and risk management; Chapter 4: Anesthesia.

Perioperative Standards and Recommended Practices. (2013), Recommended practices:
* Managing the patient receiving moderate sedation/analgesia.
* Medication safety.

Berry and Kohn's Operating Room Technique. (2013, 12th ed.), Chapter 2: Foundations of perioperative patient care standards; Chapter 23: Surgical pharmacology; Chapter 24: Anesthesia: Techniques and agents; Chapter 25: Coordinated roles of the scrub person and the circulating nurse.

Competency for Safe Patient Care During Operative and Invasive Procedures. (2009), Chapter 12: Administer drugs and solutions.

Key Words

Action, analgesia, anesthetic, cricoid pressure, delivery, documentation, drugs, seven rights, labeling, medication, medication reconciliation, moderate sedation, patient safety, pharmacology, physical status classification, physiologic response, solutions

Activity — Matching

1. Draw a line between the physical status classification and the corresponding patient.

PI   64-year-old female, history of hypertension; typically runs 150/90 to 165/100 mmHg with medication

P2   72-year-old male, diabetes mellitus type II, COPD, on dialysis and oxygen 2L/min nasal cannula

P3   86-year-old female, multisystem trauma from head-on motor vehicle accident

P4   25-year-old male, healthy, taking no medications

P5   48-year-old male, diabetes mellitus type II, takes Glyburide. Hemoglobin A1c is 6.9

2. Circle the patients who are appropriate for nurse-monitored moderate sedation.

Activity — Critical Thinking

1. You are caring for an 18-month-old patient undergoing bilateral myringotomy with insertion of ear tubes. The surgeon asks you to give an acetaminophen (Tylenol) suppository. The child weighs 26 pounds. The dose is 10 mg/kg, and the drug is supplied in 80, 120, and 325 mg suppositories.

    A. What is the correct route and dosage for this drug for this patient?

        120 / Rectal

    B. What else will you need to do to correctly administer this drug?

        Gloves, lube, ✓ ID

2. You work in a cardiac cath lab and frequently monitor patients undergoing moderate sedation/anesthesia. What monitoring equipment should be provided for safe patient care?   *BP, O2Sat, EKG*

        CO2 if poss

Activity — Do You Know?

You are monitoring a patient undergoing a central venous catheter insertion under moderate sedation. The surgeon asks you to give an initial dose of 3 mg of midazolam (Versed) IV push. You would (circle the correct response):

A. Question the surgeon. The amount is lower than the normal range for the initial recommended dose.

B. Question the surgeon. The amount is higher than the normal range for the initial recommended dose.

C. Give the dose. It is within the normal range for the initial recommended dose.

Case Study Activity

Based on Mrs. M.'s history, which anesthetic(s) should be avoided?

Halothane, Isoflurane, Enflurane, Sevoflurane, Desflurane & Succinylcholine

☆ Have MH cart avail. ✓ Dantrolene supply ☆

Activity — Short Answer

You are caring for a patient scheduled for a laparoscopic Nissen fundoplication. When you arrive to interview the patient, you find him sitting up at a 45-degree angle. He states that when he lies flat, he "gets terrible heartburn." What is the risk for this patient in undergoing a general anesthetic? What can you anticipate the anesthesiologist will need? *Aspiration / Cricoid pressure*

"Go To" Activity — Check It Out!

Go to Question #2, Medication administration; Question #5, Moderate sedation; Question #19, Pharmacology; Question #32, Propofol; and Question #41, Routine discontinuance of aspirin preoperatively, under the Perioperative question of the week tab on your CD for additional critical-thinking activities.

"Go To" Activity — Skill Building

Ask your anesthesia provider to provide an in-service, nursing grand rounds, or brown bag on safe practices for the anesthetized patient.

Review your policy on moderate sedation/analgesia and compare it with AORN's recommended practices.

Consult your state board of nursing related to nursing administration of anesthetic drugs.

Review contents of your difficult airway cart or supply box.

Additional Reading/Resources

Hicks, R.W., Wanzer, L., & Goeckner, B. (2011). Perioperative pharmacology: A framework for perioperative medication safety. *AORN Journal, 93*(1), 136-145.

Johnson, J. (2008). The increasing incidence of anesthetic adverse events in late afternoon surgeries. *AORN Journal, 88*(1), 79-87.

Mainer, J.A. (2010). Nonpharmacological interventions for assisting the induction of anesthesia in children. *AORN Journal, 92*(2), 209-210.

Mayne, I.P., & Bagaoisan, C. (2009). Social support during anesthesia induction in an adult surgical population. *AORN Journal, 89*(2), 307-320.

Wanzer, L., Goeckner, B., & Hicks, R.W. (2011). Perioperative pharmacology: Antibiotic administration. *AORN Journal, 93*(3), 340-351.

Module 3: Incorporate Principles of Safe Positioning

Every patient is positioned to afford the surgeon optimal exposure to the surgical site. This crucial step in the procedure carries with it a host of risks and potential complications, which the perioperative nurse must anticipate and work with the anesthesia provider and surgeon to prevent.

Competency Outcomes

To successfully complete the activities in this module, you will need to be able to:

1. Describe complications associated with surgical positioning.
2. Select appropriate positioning devices.
3. Choose the correct position based on procedural and patient needs.

Recommended Readings

Alexander's Care of the Patient in Surgery. (2011, 14th ed.), Chapter 2: Patient safety and risk management; Chapter 5: Positioning the patient for surgery.

Perioperative Standards and Recommended Practices. (2013), Recommended practices: Positioning the patient.

Berry and Kohn's Operating Room Technique. (2013, 12th ed.), Chapter 2: Foundations of perioperative patient care standards; Chapter 26: Positioning, prepping, and draping the patient.

Competency for Safe Patient Care During Operative and Invasive Procedures. (2009), Chapter 8: Position the patient.

Key Words

Braden score, Fowler, lateral, lithotomy, nerve injury, positioning, pressure points, prone, reverse Trendelenburg, semi-Fowler, supine, skin integrity, Trendelenburg

Activity — X Marks the Spot

Mark with an "X" the corresponding pressure points associated with the following patient positions.

Supine

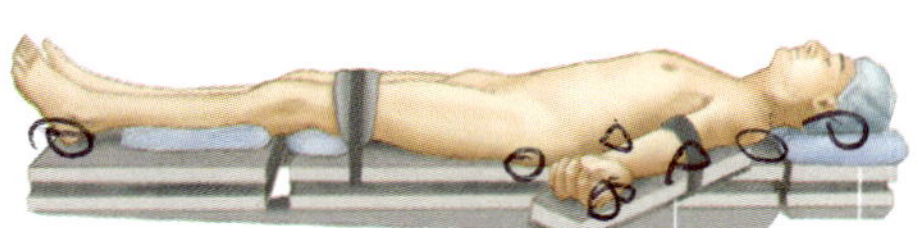

Prone

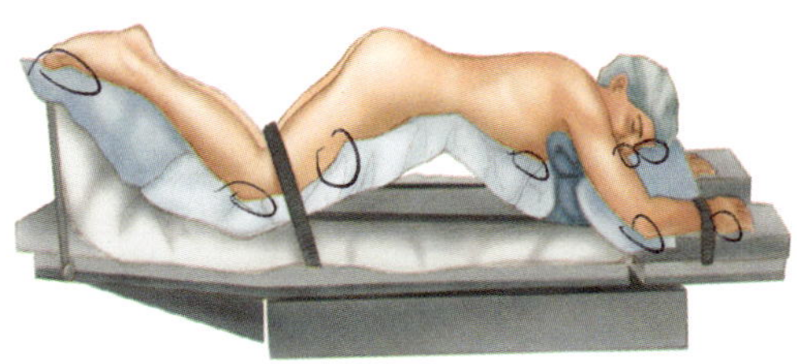

Lithotomy, boot stirrups

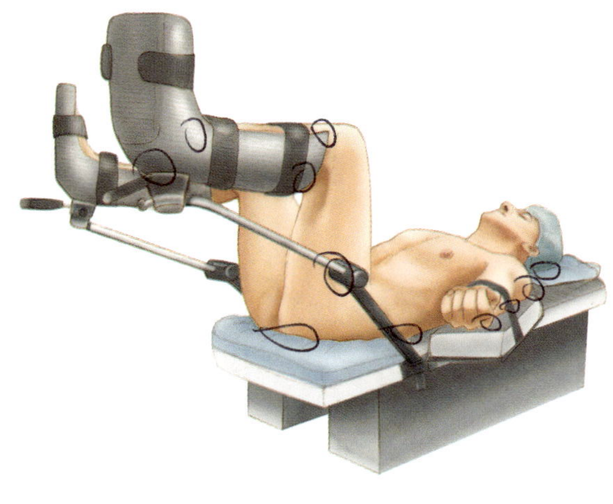

Sitting

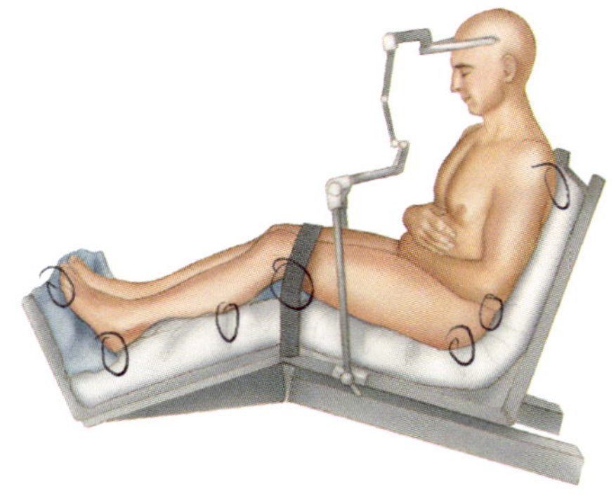

Lateral decubitis

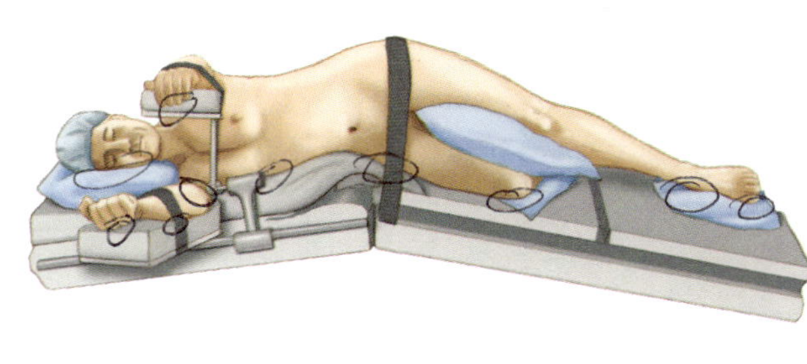

Activity — Circle the Correct Answer

In the left lateral decubitis position, the patient is lying on the _________________ side.

RIGHT   (LEFT)

Activity — Matching

Match the position with the associated nerve injury.
Answers may be used more than once.

Supine __A, E__

Lithotomy __B, C__

Lateral __A, B__

Prone __A c̄ F__

Semi-Fowler ___A___

Fowler ___E___

A. brachial plexus

B. peroneal

C. saphenous

D. sciatic

E. ulnar

F. radial

Activity — Do You Know?

The preferred placement for the patient's arms in the prone position is _____________.
(circle one)

ON ARMBOARDS   (AT THE PATIENT'S SIDES)

> ## "Go To" Activity — Skill Building
>
> Locate and review your manufacturers' manuals on the use of positioning devices.
>
> Access your facility's OR bed training manual/video or ask your industry representative to provide this information.

Additional Reading/Resources

"Go To" Activity — Check It Out!

Go to Question #40, Lithotomy positioning, under the Perioperative question of the week tab on your CD for an additional critical-thinking activity.

Bennicoff, G. (2010). Perioperative care of the morbidly obese patient in the lithotomy position. *AORN Journal, 92*(3), 297-312.

Denholm, B. (2009). Tucking patients' arms and general positioning. *AORN Journal, 89*(4), 755-757.

Munro, C.A. (2010). The development of a pressure ulcer risk-assessment scale for perioperative patients. *AORN Journal, 92*(3), 272-287.

Sewchuk, D., Padula, C., & Osborne, E. (2006). Prevention and early detection of pressure ulcers in patients undergoing cardiac surgery. *AORN Journal, 84*(1), 75-96.

St.-Arnaud D., & Paquin, M-J. (2008). Safe positioning for neurosurgical patients. *AORN Journal, 87*(6), 1156-1172.

Walton-Geer, P.S. (2009). Prevention of pressure ulcers in the surgical patient. *AORN Journal, 89*(3), 538-552.

Module 4: Prepare the Surgical Site

By definition, the surgical incision breaches one of the body's main protective barriers — the skin. Understanding and applying current best practices in patient skin preparation can decrease the risk of surgical site infections.

Competency Outcomes

To successfully complete the activities in this module, you will need to be able to:

1. Classify stages of wound healing.
2. Apply the appropriate skin preparation antiseptic based on skin integrity, number and kinds of contaminants, patient's individual needs (e.g., allergies), and area to be prepped.
3. Choose methods of hair removal based on current best practice.

Recommended Readings

Alexander's Care of the Patient in Surgery. (2011, 14th ed.), Chapter 3: Infection prevention and control in the perioperative setting.

Perioperative Standards and Recommended Practices. (2013), Recommended practices: Preoperative patient skin antisepsis.

Berry and Kohn's Operating Room Technique. (2013, 12th ed.), Chapter 26: Positioning, prepping, and draping the patient.

Competency for Safe Patient Care During Operative and Invasive Procedures. (2009), Chapter 5: Preparation of the patient for the procedure; Chapter 9: Establish and maintain the sterile field.

Key Words

Antiseptic, cleansing, prep, skin antisepsis, surgical site

Activity — Critical Thinking

You are caring for a patient who is scheduled for reanastomosis of a colostomy. How is the typical skin prep adjusted for this patient?

Do colostomy site last. Prep around 1st. Can put betadine soaked gauze on. Don't prep colostomy c̄ chloraprep / duraprep.

Activity — Critical Thinking

The surgeon requests that hair be removed from the immediate incisional area for an extremely hirsute male scheduled for an inguinal herniorraphy. What is the best method for accomplishing this? *Clippers*

> ## "Go To" Activity — Check It Out!
>
> Go to Question #3, Prepping agents for mucous membranes, and Question #35, Shellfish and prep agents, under the Perioperative question of the week tab on your CD for additional critical-thinking activities.

Activity — Color Me

For each illustration on the following pages, mark the incision (if applicable) and shade the area to be prepped.

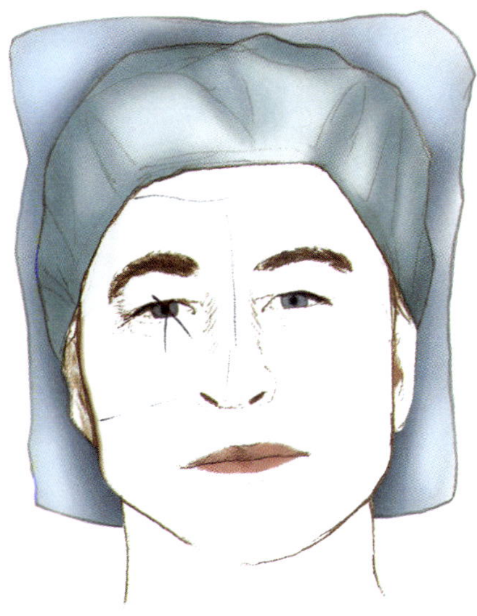

Cataract extraction, right eye

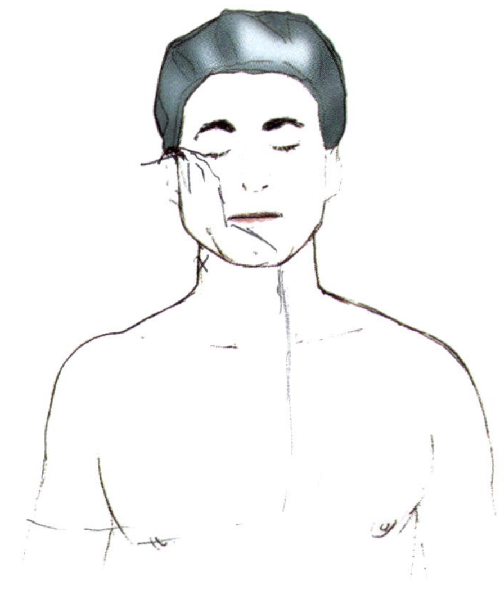

Right carotid endarterectomy

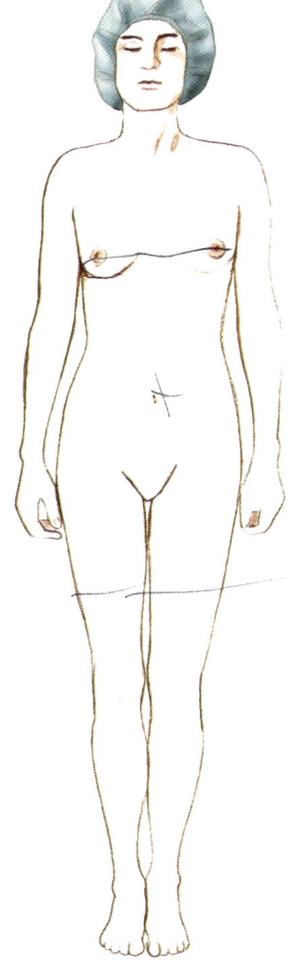

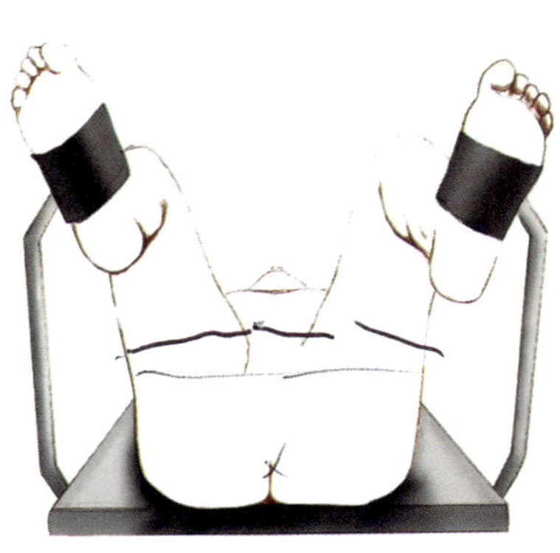

Abdominal/perineal resection

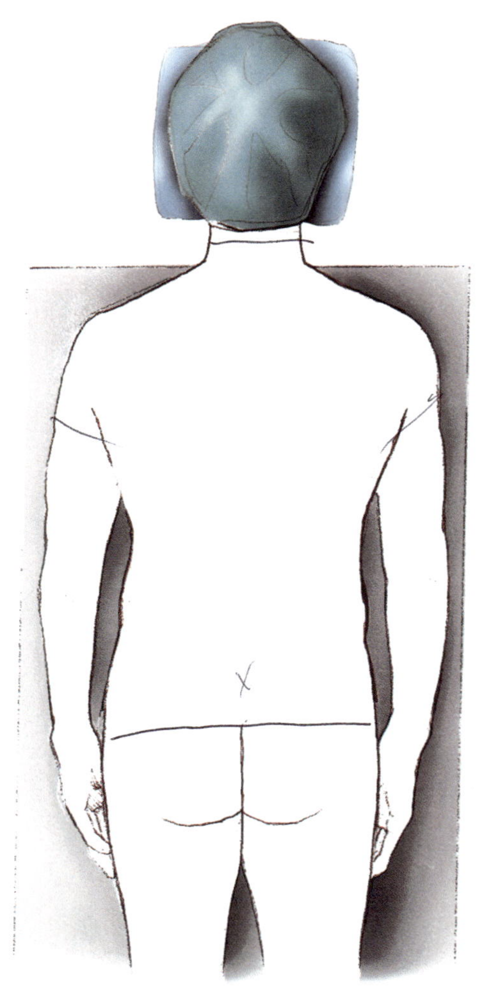

Lumbar discectomy, L4-L5

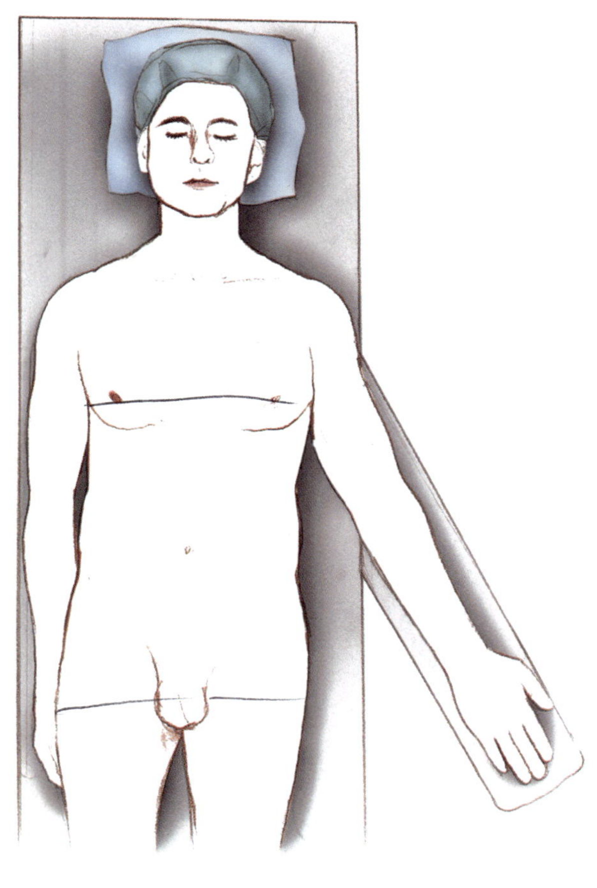

Laparoscopic cholecystectomy

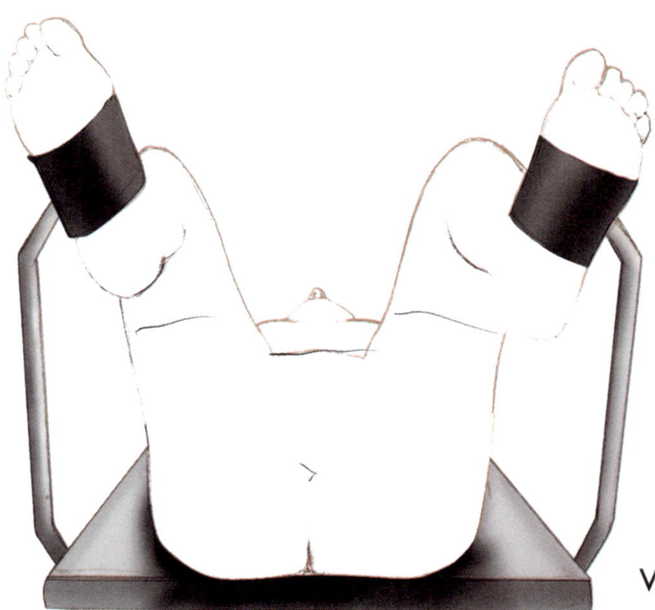

Vaginal hysterectomy

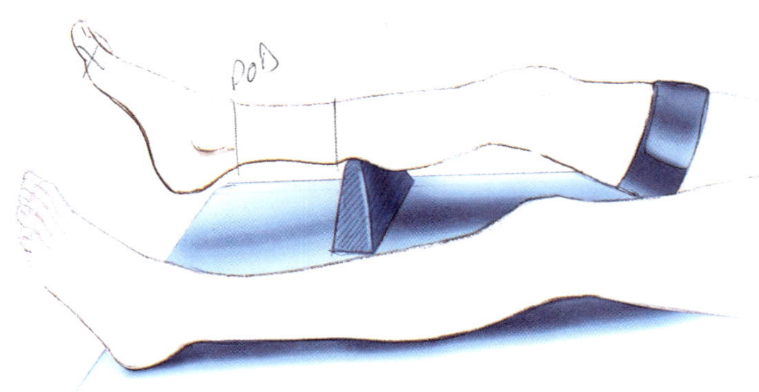

Right bunionectomy

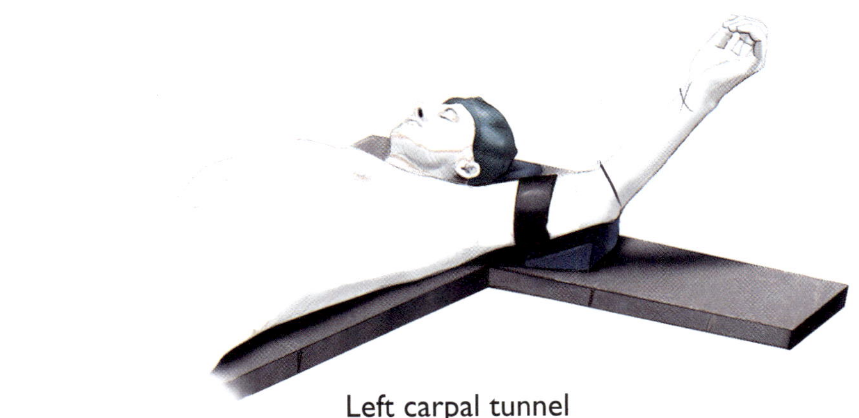

Left carpal tunnel

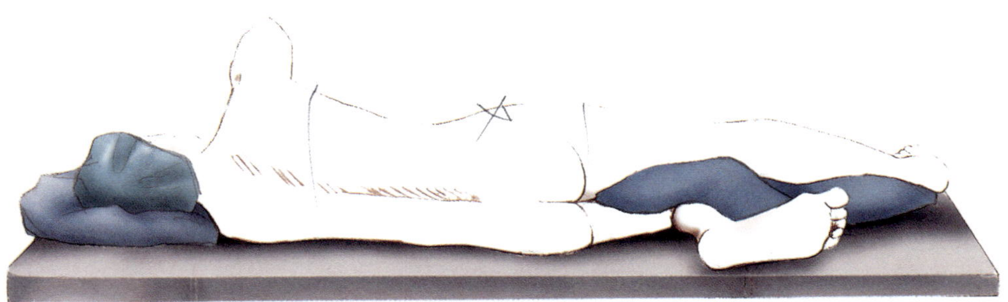

Right nephrectomy

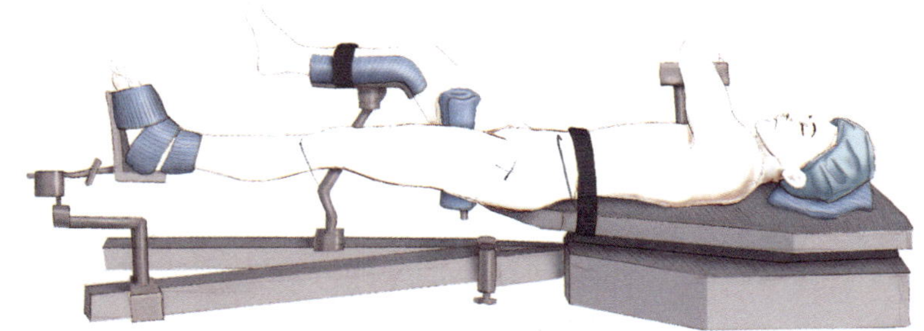

Left hip arthroplasty

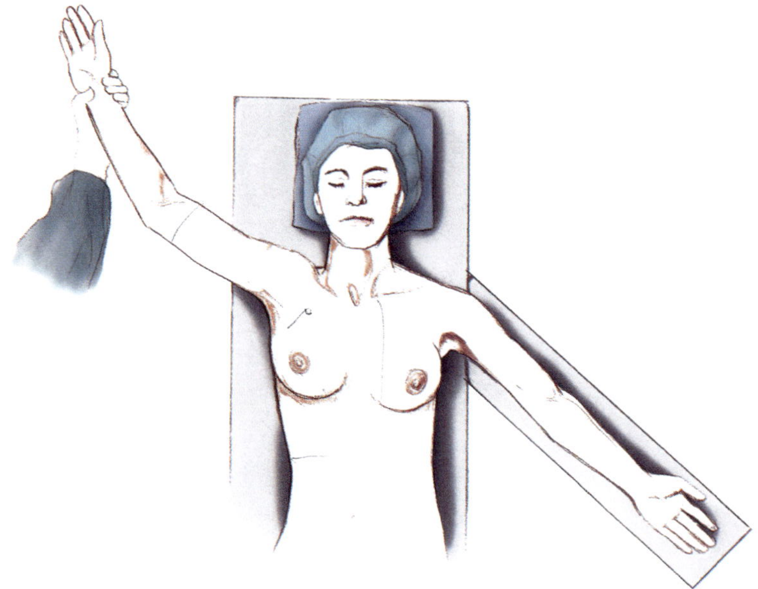

Right lumpectomy, right upper quadrant

"Go To" Activity — Skill Building

Compare your facility's policy and procedure related to patient skin preparation with AORN's recommended practices on patient skin antisepsis.

Additional Reading/Resources

DeBaun, B. (2008). Evaluation of the antimicrobial properties of an alcohol-free 2% chlorhexidine gluconate solution. *AORN Journal, 87*(5), 925-933.

Edmiston, C. E., Okoli, O., Graham, M.B., Sinski, S., et al. (2010). Evidence for using chlorhexidine gluconate preoperative cleansing to reduce the risk of surgical site infection. *AORN Journal, 92*(5), 509-518.

Grelle, K., Linker, L., Maninang, J., Bruce, S., et al. (2008). Standardization of a surgical site precleansing technique for vascular patients. *AORN Journal, 88*(2), 261-265.

Institute for Healthcare Improvement (IHI). (2013). Prevent surgical site infection. Retrieved Feb. 4, 2013, from http://www.ihi.org/explore/SSI/Pages/default.aspx.

Zinn, J., Jenkins, J.B., Swofford, V., Harrelson, B., et al. (2010). Intraoperative patient skin prep agents: Is there a difference? *AORN Journal, 92*(6), 662-674.

Module 5: Apply Principles of Asepsis

Observing the basic rules of asepsis is the most important action the perioperative nurse can perform in helping to prevent surgical site infections. In addition to being responsible for his/her own actions, the nurse's strong sense of surgical conscience implies holding all members of the surgical care team to those same high standards.

Competency Outcomes

To successfully complete the activities in this module, you will need to be able to:

1. Apply principles of asepsis to perioperative nursing actions.
2. Identify actions to correct breaks in technique.
3. Classify wounds according to Centers for Disease Control and Prevention definitions.

Recommended Readings

Alexander's Care of the Patient in Surgery. (2011, 14th ed.), Chapter 2: Patient safety and risk management; Chapter 3: Infection prevention and control in the perioperative setting.

Perioperative Standards and Recommended Practices. (2013), Recommended practices:
- Surgical attire.
- Hand hygiene.
- Sterile technique.
- Traffic patterns.
- Product selection.
- Prevention of transmissible infections.

Berry and Kohn's Operating Room Technique. (2013, 12th ed.), Chapter 2: Foundations of perioperative patient care standards; Chapter 15: Principles of asepsis and sterile techniques; Chapter 16: Appropriate attire, surgical hand cleansing, gowning, and gloving; Chapter 20: Wound healing and hemostasis, p. 577.

Competency for Safe Patient Care During Operative and Invasive Procedures. (2009), Chapter 9: Establish and maintain the sterile field.

Key Words

Asepsis, gloving, gowning, hand hygiene, sterile field, sterile technique, surgical attire, surgical consciousness, traffic patterns

Activity — Matching

Match the area with the required appropriate attire. Answers may be used more than once.

Cafeteria _____ *E*

Sterile supply room *B, C, D*

OR with opened supplies *A, B, C, D*

A. mask
B. surgical scrubs
C. hair covering
D. coverall/jumpsuit
E. street clothes

Activity — Fill In the Blank

For the following procedures, write in the corresponding wound classification:

Total knee replacement: _____ *clean (1)*

Incision and drainage of abscess, status postop posterior spinal fusion: *infected (4)*

Appendectomy, unruptured: *clean/contaminated (2)*

Open reduction internal fixation open fracture right radius/ulna: *contaminated (3)*

Activity — Short Answer

1. You are turning over your room for a cystoscopy for a 7-year-old girl. You drop an unopened box of 4X4 radiopaque sponges on the floor. What should you do?

Toss

2. You are scrubbed for a lumpectomy for a 44-year-old woman. The surgeon asks you to move to the other side of the table to hold a retractor. What is the appropriate way to pass the other scrubbed members of the team?

Back to back

"Go To" Activity — Check It Out!

Go to Question #15, Surgical attire, and Question #16, Infection control, under the Perioperative question of the week tab on your CD for critical-thinking questions.

Additional Reading/Resources

Blanchard, J. (2009). Reuse of multidose vials. *AORN Journal, 89*(6), 1128-1129.

Chard, R. (2008). Clinical Issues: Wound classifications. *AORN Journal, 88*(1), 108-109.

Hopper, W.R., & Moss, R. (2010). Common breaks in sterile technique: Clinical perspectives and perioperative implications. *AORN Journal, 91*(3), 350-367.

Module 6: Provide Perioperative Nursing Care During Operative and Invasive Procedures

The CNOR exam contains questions related to many different procedures and patient types, some of which may not be familiar to you; therefore, it is highly recommended that you take advantage of opportunities to care for as many different types of patients and procedures as possible in your work setting. Providing examples of every specialty is beyond the scope of this book. By completing the activities, however, you have been provided with the tools to develop your own plan of care for any patient.

Competency Outcomes

To successfully complete the activities in this module, you will need to be able to:

1. Relate pertinent anatomy and physiology to the proposed procedure.
2. Organize a plan of care to accommodate surgical and patient needs.
3. Anticipate and prevent complications inherent to surgery.

Recommended Readings

Alexander's Care of the Patient in Surgery. (2011, 14th ed.), Chapter 3: Infection prevention and control in the perioperative setting; Chapter 6: Sutures, needles, and instruments; Chapter 7: Surgical modalities; Chapter 8: Wound healing, dressings, and drains; Unit II: Surgical interventions; Unit III: Special considerations.

Perioperative Standards and Recommended Practices. (2013), Recommended practices:
- Minimally invasive surgery.
- Surgical tissue banking.
- Managing the patient receiving local anesthesia.
- Managing the patient receiving moderate sedation/analgesia.

Berry and Kohn's Operating Room Technique. (2013, 12th ed.), Chapter 19: Surgical instrumentation; Chapter 25: Coordinated roles of the scrub person and the circulating nurse; Chapter 28: Surgical incisions, implants, and wound closure; Chapter 29: Wound healing and hemostasis; Chapter 31: Potential perioperative complications; Section 12: Surgical specialties.

Competency for Safe Patient Care During Operative and Invasive Procedures. (2009), Chapter 16: Handle tissue with instruments; Chapter 17: Provide hemostasis; Section III: Operative and invasive procedures; Section IV: Age specific care.

Key Words

Anatomy, hemostasis, implant, invasive procedure, minimally invasive, operation, physiology, specialty, surgery, wound healing

"Go To" Case Study Activity

From your previously developed concept map and the patient assessment, develop a plan of care for the intraoperative component of Mrs. M.'s perioperative experience.

1. Identify the intraoperative nursing interventions that will need to be implemented for Mrs. M.'s surgical procedure. Some of these are typical for every surgery (e.g., infection prevention, principles of aseptic technique, skin antisepsis), while others will be specific for Mrs. M.

2. Arrange the intraoperative activities from your list under their corresponding "major problems" boxes you developed in Chapters 1 and 2.

3. What critical information needs to be communicated to the following health care team members?

Anesthesia provider:

Surgeon:

Scrub person:

PACU:

Activity — Short Answer

A 17-year-old patient returns to your facility seven months postoperatively for removal of an infected Harrington rod implant. The wound cultures *Staphylococcus aureus*. Is this considered a surgical site infection? Why or why not?

Activity — Name That Incision

Name the abdominal incisions in the diagram below.

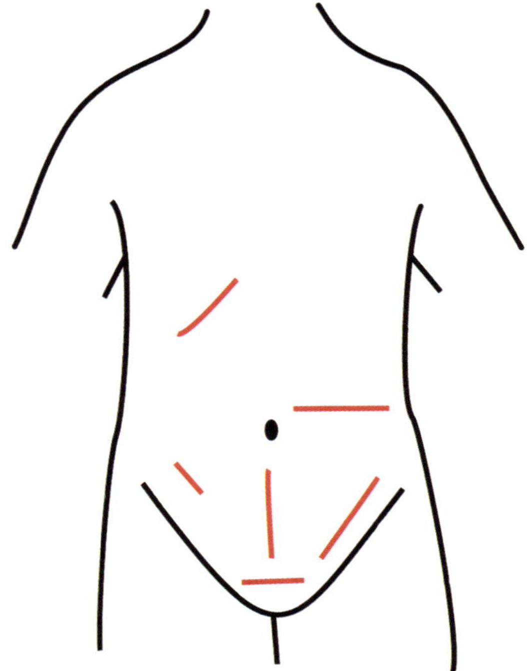

Activity — Matching

Match the incision types listed above to their corresponding surgical procedure. Use each answer only once.

Lower midline _______

Oblique _______

Pfannenstiel _______

Subcostal _______

McBurney _______

Transverse _______

A. abdominal hysterectomy

B. appendectomy

C. radical retropubic prostatectomy

D. open inguinal herniorraphy

E. hepatic resection

F. choledochojejunostomy

Activity — Short Answer

Your patient is scheduled for an ulnar nerve release, left elbow; he states that he has an implantable cardiodefibrillator. What is the safest electrosurgical method to use, and why?

Additional Reading/Resources

Note: Every *AORN Journal* typically includes at least one article on a surgical specialty.

Doerflinger, D.M.C. (2009). Older adult surgical patients: Presentation and challenges. *AORN Journal, 90*(2), 223-244.

Harrington, S., Simmons, K., Thomas, C., & Scully, S. (2008). Pediatric laparoscopy. *AORN Journal, 88*(2), 211-240.

Ide, P., Farber, E.S., & Lautz, D. (2008). Perioperative nursing care of the bariatric surgical patient. *AORN Journal, 88*(1), 30-58.

Ulmer, B. (2010). Best practices for minimally invasive procedures. *AORN Journal, 91*(5), 558-575.

Module 7: Identify and Control Environmental Factors

Managing intraoperative environmental factors (e.g., temperature, humidity, traffic flow, noise) contributes to optimal patient outcomes. The push for shorter turnover times should not compromise room cleaning, which is frequently performed by unlicensed assistive personnel with limited knowledge of transmission of infectious agents or antiseptic principles. It is ultimately the perioperative nurse's responsibility to ensure that the intraoperative environment is safe and meets facility and regulatory standards for providing safe patient care.

Competency Outcomes

To successfully complete the activities in this module, you will need to be able to:

1. Select normal values for air exchanges, humidity, and temperature.
2. Apply principles of antisepsis to maintenance of a clean environment.

Recommended Readings

Alexander's Care of the Patient in Surgery. (2011, 14th ed.), Chapter 3: Infection prevention and control in the perioperative setting; Chapter 4: Anesthesia.

AORN. (2009). Position statement on noise in the perioperative practice setting. Retrieved Feb. 4, 2013, from http://www.aorn.org/Clinical_Practice/Position_Statements/Position_Statements. aspx.

Perioperative Standards and Recommended Practices. (2012), Recommended practices:
- Environmental cleaning in the perioperative setting.
- Safe environment of care.

Berry and Kohn's Operating Room Technique. (2013, 12th ed.), Chapter 10: Physical facilities; Chapter 11: Ambulatory surgery centers and alternative surgery locations; Chapter 12: Care of the intraoperative environment; Chapter 13: Potential sources of injury to the caregiver and the patient.

Competency for Safe Patient Care During Operative and Invasive Procedures. (2009), Chapter 14: Monitor and control the environment.

Key Words

Air exchanges, antiseptic, environmental cleaning, humidity, infectious waste, noise, room turnover, spills, temperature, terminal cleaning, traffic patterns, turnover

Activity — Fill In the Blank

For each of the following environmental controls, list the acceptable parameters:

Air exchanges:

OR:_________ Cardiac cath lab:_________ Sterile storage area: _________
Decontamination area: _________

Humidity:

OR:_________ Cardiac cath lab:_________ Decontamination area: _________

Temperature:

OR:_________ Cardiac cath lab:_________ Decontamination area: _________

Air pressure in the OR should be _________________ than the surrounding corridors.
(greater/lower)

Activity — Short Answer

For each source of noise, list a nursing intervention to reduce its risk of disrupting the environment and impacting patient safety:

Beeper/pager/cell phone:

Monitor alarms:

Electronic music devices (radios, CD players):

Overhead pages and announcements:

Telephones:

Staff communication:

Case Study Activity

As the anesthesia care provider hands you a tube of blood for a blood chemistry analysis for Mrs. M., it slips out of your hand and drops to the floor, breaking the tube. What is the best way to clean up the spill?

"Go To" Activity — Skill Building

Compare how your facility monitors and documents OR air exchange rates, temperature, and humidity with AORN standards and recommended practices.

"Go To" Activity — Check It Out!

Go to Question #11, Infection Control, under the Perioperative question of the week tab on your CD for a critical-thinking question related to cleaning a room after a patient infected with MRSA.

Activity — Critical Thinking

How does end of procedure (turnover) cleaning between cases differ from that done at the end of the day (terminal cleaning)?

Additional Readings/Resources

Blanchard, J. (2009). Terminal cleaning. *AORN Journal, 89*(2), 409-411.

Jefferson, J., Whelan, R., Dick, B., & Carling, P. (2011). A novel technique for identifying opportunities to improve environmental hygiene in the operating room. *AORN Journal, 93*(3), 358-364.

Module 8: Monitor and Intervene to Reduce the Risk of Complications and Adverse Outcomes

A variety of equipment unique to the OR contributes to maintaining the high level of technologically sophisticated care enjoyed by today's surgical patient. This same equipment also holds inherent risks that must be safely managed to avoid injury to both patients and staff.

Competency Outcomes

To successfully complete the activities in this module, you will need to be able to:

1. Identify common hazards associated with the intraoperative environment.
2. Recognize the importance of following manufacturers' recommendations for safely operating their equipment.

Recommended Readings

Alexander's Care of the Patient in Surgery. (2011, 14th ed.), Chapter 2: Patient safety and risk management; Chapter 30: Workplace issues and staff safety.

Perioperative Standards and Recommended Practices. (2013), Recommended practices:
- Electrosurgery.
- Laser safety in practice settings.
- Pneumatic tourniquet.
- Reducing radiological exposure.

AORN. (2011). Position statement: Creating a practice environment of safety. Retrieved Feb. 21, 2013, from http://www.aorn.org/Clinical_Practice/Position_Statements/Position_Statements.aspx

Perioperative Standards and Recommended Practices. (2013), Guidance statement:
- Sharps injury prevention.

Berry and Kohn's Operating Room Technique. (2013, 12th ed.), Chapter 2: Foundations of perioperative patient care standards; Chapter 13: Potential sources of injury to the caregiver and patient; Chapter 20: Specialized surgical equipment; Chapter 22: Diagnostic procedures and oncologic considerations; Chapter 27: Physiologic maintenance and monitoring of the perioperative patient; Chapter 31: Potential perioperative complications.

Competency for Safe Patient Care During Operative and Invasive Procedures. (2009), Chapter 14: Monitor and control the environment.

Key Words

Adverse event, body mechanics, chemicals, electrosurgery, ergonomics, equipment testing, fire, laser, National Patient Safety Goals, radiation, patient safety, sharps injury, smoke evacuation

Activity — Fill in the Blank

The three principles related to radiation protection are _____________________________,

_____________________________, and _____________________________.

Activity — Critical Thinking

1. You are the circulating nurse for an 11-year-old boy undergoing an open reduction internal fixation for a right malleolar fracture from a skate-board accident. You notice that the tourniquet time is approaching 60 minutes. What should you do?

2. Your patient is scheduled for a laser tonsillectomy. What safety mechanisms should be in place to care for your patient?

Case Study Activity

1. Back injuries are one of the most frequently cited occupational injuries for health care workers. What interventions can you implement to transfer Mrs. M. safely during her perioperative experience?

2. Dr. S. has called for an intraoperative cholangiogram for Mrs. M. What protective measures need to be implemented to protect Mrs. M. and the staff in the room?

3. Dr. S. repeatedly asks for the coagulation power on the electrosurgical unit to be increased. You know that a need for abnormally high settings may indicate a problem with the system. What steps should be taken in trouble-shooting a possible problem?

4. Upon completion of the surgery, a slightly reddened area is noted on Mrs. M.'s left thigh under the electrosurgical dispersive electrode. As her nurse, what steps do you need to take to document this incident?

"Go To" Activity — Skill Building

Talk with your facility quality department or laser safety officer about the most current safety standards regarding use of lasers in your facility.

Compare your policy on laser use with AORN's recommended practices.

Check with your industry representative who supplies your electrosurgical equipment and supplies for educational materials on dispersive electrode safety and adverse effects of surgical smoke plume exposure.

Ask the radiation safety officer at your facility to provide a staff in-service to discuss patient and staff radiation safety issues, including what staff can do to promote safe practices when exposed to radiation in the OR. Ask for information on the proper way to wear monitoring badges based on facility and state standards.

Ask your risk mitigation officer to review your facility's policy on occurrence reporting.

Additional Reading/Resources

Blanchard, J. (2009). Protecting personnel who work with radiation. *AORN Journal, 89*(6), 1127-1128.

Edwards, B.E., & Reiman, R.E. (2008). Results of a survey on current surgical smoke control practices. *AORN Journal, 87*(4), 739-749.

Smith, F.D. (2010). Management of exposure to waste anesthetic gases. *AORN Journal, 91*(4), 482-494.

Vose, J.G,. & Adara-Berkowitz, J. (2009). Reducing scalpel injuries in the operating room. *AORN Journal, 90*(6), 867-872.

Watson, D. (2010). Radiation safety. *AORN Journal, 92*(2), 233-235.

Watson, D. (2010). Surgical smoke evacuation during laparoscopic surgery. *AORN Journal, 92*(3), 347-350.

Module 9: Prepare and Label Specimens

Although tissue, body fluids, and bone typically come to mind when specimens are discussed, a specimen is anything removed from a patient's body. In addition to assisting in providing a diagnosis, the results of specimen analysis may influence the course of treatment, the need for additional procedures, and forensic evidence.

Competency Outcomes

To successfully complete the activities in this module, you will need to be able to:

1. Prepare a specimen for transport to the laboratory.
2. Describe items to include in identification of a specimen.

Recommended Readings

Alexander's Care of the Patient in Surgery. (2011, 14th ed.), Chapter 2: Patient safety and risk management.

Perioperative Standards and Recommended Practices. (2013), Recommended practices: Care and handling of specimens in the perioperative environment.

Berry and Kohn's Operating Room Technique. (2013, 12th ed.), Chapter 2: Foundations of perioperative patient care standards, p. 26: Chapter 22: Diagnostics, specimens, and oncologic considerations; Chapter 25: Coordinated roles of the scrub person and the circulating nurse.

Competency for Safe Patient Care During Operative and Invasive Procedures. (2009), Chapter 15: Handle specimens and cultures.

Key Words

Culture, documentation, explanted medical device, handling, implanted medical device, specimen, tissue tracking

Activity — Short Answer

Identification of the specimen should be confirmed verbally between the circulating nurse and the surgeon using a "read back" communication similar to that used with verbal orders. What information needs to be communicated between the surgeon and circulating nurse?

Activity — True or False

1. Formalin is considered a hazardous chemical that should be disposed of according to OSHA regulations.

TRUE   FALSE

2. The specimen label should be placed on the lid of the container.

TRUE   FALSE

<table>
<tr><td>

"Go To" Activity — Skill Building

Take a field trip to your laboratory. Ask to observe how different tissues are processed.

Review your facility's policy on processing explanted medical devices; how does it differ from AORN recommended practices?

</td><td>

"Go To" Activity — Check It Out!

Go to Question #14, Specimen handling, and Question #31, Forensics, under the Perioperative question of the week tab on your CD for critical-thinking activities.

</td></tr>
</table>

Module 10: Perform Counts

Retained surgical items (RSIs) cause unnecessary pain and suffering to the patient and additional expense to the health care facility. RSIs are considered a sentinel or "never event" and are required to be reported to The Joint Commission. A primary goal of performing counts is to avoid RSIs by providing consistent, standardized, and achievable methods for accounting for suture, instruments, and sharps.

Competency Outcomes

To successfully complete the activities in this module, you will need to be able to:

1. Identify appropriate items to be counted at the correct time.
2. Describe the correct action to take for an incorrect count.

Recommended Readings

Alexander's Care of the Patient in Surgery. (2011, 14th ed.), Chapter 2: Patient safety and risk management; Chapter 6: Sutures, needles, and instruments.

Perioperative Standards and Recommended Practices. (2013), Recommended practices: Prevention of retained surgical items.

Berry and Kohn's Operating Room Technique. (2013, 12th ed.), Chapter 2: Foundations of perioperative patient care standards; Chapter 25: Coordinated roles of the scrub person and the circulating nurse.

Competency for Safe Patient Care During Operative and Invasive Procedures. (2009), Chapter 10: Perform sponge, sharp, and instrument counts.

Key Words

Closing, complication, count, instruments, needles, retained item, sharps, sponges

Activity — Do You Know?

How many strategies can you list to help prevent a retained surgical item?

Activity — Critical Thinking

You are counting sponges with the scrub person in preparation for an abdominal hysterectomy. The package of 4X4 radiopaque sponges you have opened contains 9 sponges instead of 10. What should you do?

Activity — Scramble

Number the following steps in the correct order for completing a sponge and suture count:

______ When wound (peritoneum) closure begins

______ Before the procedure

______ At skin closure

______ Before closure of a cavity (e.g., uterus or bladder) within a cavity

List two other circumstances when a count should be performed:

1.__________________________________   2.__________________________________

Case Study Activity

Mrs. M.'s surgery is near completion. As a needle holder and needle were returned to the scrub person, he noted that the needle was bent with the tip of the needle missing. Explain your immediate course of action to prevent a retained surgical item. How would you document these issues and the patient care you provided?

"Go To" Activity Check It Out!	**"Go To" Activity — Skill Building**
Go to Question #1, Counts, under the Perioperative question of the week tab on your CD for a critical-thinking question.	Compare your facility's policy and procedure on preventing retained items to AORN's standards and recommended practices. Ask your risk mitigation manager to provide an in-service on the tools used to investigate an event related to a retained surgical item, e.g., root cause analysis (RCA), failure mode effects analysis (FMEA), etc.

Additional Reading/Resources

Edel, E. M. (2010). Increasing patient safety and surgical team communication by using a count/time out board. *AORN Journal, 92*(4), 420-424.

Jackson, S., & Brady, S. (2008). Counting difficulties: Retained instruments, sponges, and needles. *AORN Journal, 87*(2), 315-321.

Mitchell, S. (2009). Placing count sheets in instrument trays. *AORN Journal, 90*(2), 280-281.

Pelter, M.M., Stephens, K.E., & Loranger, D. (2007). An evaluation of a numbered surgical sponge product. *AORN Journal, 85*(5), 931-940.

Rowland, A., & Steeves, R. (2010). Incorrect sponge counts: A qualitative analysis. *AORN Journal, 92*(4), 410-419.

Module 11: Maintain Accurate Patient Records

Many medical errors are due to incomplete or inaccurately documented patient data. One of the goals behind the current movement to record patient information electronically is to provide a standardized framework for documenting data that makes it more difficult to input information incorrectly or not at all. Regardless of the method used, maintenance of accurate patient information related to the surgical experience requires careful attention to detail and should go beyond "checking the boxes." In addition to providing a history of the patient's intraoperative experience, this information will be used as a reference for other health care providers; for quality improvement projects and billing; for reordering of implants, prostheses, and supplies; as a measure of meeting benchmarks for regulatory surveys; and as evidence in a court of law.

Competency Outcomes

To successfully complete the activities in this module, you will need to be able to:

1. Identify data elements to be included in an intraoperative patient record.
2. Use information found in patient records to improve quality of care.

Recommended Readings

Alexander's Care of the Patient in Surgery. (2011, 14th ed.), Chapter 2: Patient safety and risk management.

Perioperative Standards and Recommended Practices. (2013), Recommended practices: Information management.

Berry and Kohn's Operating Room Technique. (2013, 12th ed.), Chapter 2: Foundations of perioperative patient care standards; Chapter 3: Legal, regulatory, and ethical issues; Chapter 11: Ambulatory surgery centers and alternative surgical locations; Chapter 25: Coordinated roles of the scrub person and the circulating nurse.

Competency for Safe Patient Care During Operative and Invasive Procedures. (2009), Chapter 6: Transfer the patient; Chapter 10: Perform sponge, sharp, and instrument counts.

Key Words

Confidentiality, documentation, electronic medical record (EMR), patient record

Activity — Critical Thinking

You work in a free-standing ambulatory surgery center that enjoys a thriving plastic surgery practice. Your facility has just received a letter from the FDA recalling a certain brand of breast implant. What information from the patients' records do you need to have in determining which of your patients are affected by this recall?

Additional Reading/ Resources

Beach, M.J., & Sions, J.A. (2011). Surviving OR computerization. *AORN Journal, 93*(2), 226-241.

Gunn, M. (2008). Standardized perioperative record: A bold step forward. *AORN Journal, 88*(6), S66-S67.

"Go To" Activity — Skill Building

Compare your facility's patient record with the suggested examples in AORN's recommended practices. How do they differ?

Volunteer to serve on a quality improvement committee or chart audit project.

O'Meara, E. (2007). The effects of electronic documentation in the ambulatory surgery setting. *AORN Journal, 86*(6), 970-979.

Saletnik, L.A., Niedlinger, M.K., & Wilson, M. (2008). Nursing resource considerations for implementing an electronic documentation system. *AORN Journal, 87*(3), 585-596.

Chapter Summary

Caring for the patient in the intraoperative phase requires a highly developed combination of knowledge and skills that is unique to this specialty. This chapter reviewed the key aspects of intraoperative nursing activities as they relate to the safety, physical, psychological, and sociocultural issues included in the patient's surgical experience. Commitment to quality patient care by implementing current best practices is highlighted.

Glossary

AORN Perioperative Standards and Recommended Practices — As used in the Job Analysis, this term includes all sections of the *Perioperative Standards and Recommended Practices,* published annually by AORN. The most current edition should be used at all times.

Association for the Advancement of Medical Instrumentation (AAMI) — An organization with the goal of increasing the understanding and beneficial use of medical instrumentation. AAMI is the primary source of consensus and timely information on medical instrumentation and technology and is the primary resource for national and international standards for industry, professional organizations, and government agencies. (www. aami.org)

Association of periOperative Registered Nurses (AORN) — AORN is the professional organization of perioperative registered nurses that supports registered nurses in achieving optimal outcomes for patients undergoing operative and other invasive procedures. (www.aorn.org)

Centers for Disease Control and Prevention (CDC) — The federal government agency dedicated to monitoring disease, mortality, and morbidity of patients in the United States. This agency sets guidelines for dealing with known or suspected diseases. The CDC serves as the national focus for developing and applying disease prevention and control, environmental health, and health promotion and education activities designed to improve the health of the people of the United States. (www.cdc.gov)

Cultural diversity — Backgrounds, beliefs, values, and ethnicities that play a major role in communication and interactions between patients and perioperative nurses. Every patient must be evaluated for individual cultural considerations in the perioperative setting.

Delegation — The transfer of responsibility for the performance of an activity from one individual to another while retaining accountability for the outcome.

Domain (related to the PNDS) — The four overall divisions of the conceptual framework of the *Perioperative Nursing Data Set.* All interventions and expected outcomes relate to one or more domain(s). The four domains are Safety, Physiologic Responses, Behavioral Responses, and the Health System.

Healthcare Insurance Portability and Accountability Act (HIPAA) — Legislation passed in 1996 that addresses various aspects of the use of patients' medical information, including confidentiality of patient information in the medical record, consent processes for access to patients' health information, and the right to sue the health plan provider.

Hypothermia — A body temperature significantly below normal (i.e., 98.6° F [37° C]).

May be caused by the operating room environment (e.g., room temperature, exposed skin) and can interfere with patient's maintenance of a normal physiologic state.

Informed consent — The patient's right to make his or her own informed decisions based on information regarding treatment options, including the benefits, expected outcomes, and risk and potential complications; right to refuse treatment; and decisions regarding participation in research studies.

Intervention (nursing) — Action taken, based on patient assessment data, with the intention of achieving one or more expected patient outcomes.

Intraoperative phase — Begins when the patient is transferred to the operating room bed and ends when he or she is admitted to the postanesthesia care unit.

Outcome criteria — Statements developed to identify the tasks or conditions to be implemented that will assist the patient in achieving the desired outcomes. Outcome criteria indicate an expected, measurable change in the patient's health status.

Patients' rights — The rights of every patient to seek and receive health care regardless of his or her race, religion, or culture and with respect for the individual's self-image, privacy, and other such considerations, in accordance with the Patients' Bill of Rights.

Perioperative Nursing Data Set (PNDS) — The perioperative nursing vocabulary guidebook that provides nursing diagnosis, nursing interventions, and patient outcomes statements specific to the perioperative environment.

Perioperative period — Time commencing with the decision for surgical intervention and ending with a follow-up home or clinical evaluation. This period includes the preoperative, intraoperative, and postoperative phases.

Plan of care (or care plan) — A result of a systematic process of identifying expected patient outcomes and determining how to achieve them. It includes the list of interventions necessary to reach the expected outcome. The plan of care directs all nursing care activities related to each patient.

Primary intention — The desired form of wound healing, in which no tissue loss, strict adherence to aseptic technique, and close approximation of wound edges allow for optimal healing with minimal formation of scar tissue.

Regulatory standards — CDC and Occupational Safety and Health Administration regulations and standards and federal, state, and local laws and regulations that govern practice.

Safe environment — The setting in which the physical and psychological aspects of the environment are controlled for the purpose of presenting the least possible hazard to the patient, staff members, and community.

Sentinel event — An unexpected occurrence involving death or serious physical or psychological injury, or the risk thereof.

Surgical intervention — The patient's experiences during the preoperative, intraoperative, and postoperative phases, including the technical aspects and anatomical approach.

Surgical procedure — The technical aspects and anatomical approach used during surgical intervention.

Teaching and learning theories and techniques — Those aids and methods that facilitate learning (e.g., audiovisual tools, return demonstration, adult learning principles).

Terminal cleaning — Thorough cleaning and disinfection of the perioperative environment at the end of daily use.

Transfer — Moving a patient from one place to another (e.g., to or from a bed or stretcher).

Transport — Moving a patient via a device (e.g., wheelchair, stretcher).

Turnover — Cleaning and preparation of the OR between cases for the next patient's arrival.

Universal Protocol Time-Out — As an integral component of The Joint Commission's Universal Protocol for Preventing Wrong Site, Wrong Procedure, Wrong Person Surgery, time-out surgical site verification must be conducted in the location where the procedure will be done, just before starting the procedure. It must involve the entire operative team, use active communication, be briefly documented, and include, at the least
- Correct patient identity
- Correct side and site
- Agreement on the procedure to be done
- Correct patient position
- Availability of correct implants and any special equipment or requirements

Processes and systems should be in place for reconciling differences in staff responses during the time-out.

Unlicensed assistive personnel — Individuals who are trained to function in an assistive role to the registered nurse in providing patient care activities as delegated by, and under the supervision of, the registered nurse.

World Health Organization (WHO) — The directing and coordinating authority for health within the United Nations system. It is responsible for providing leadership on global health matters, shaping the health research agenda, setting norms and standards, articulating evidence-based policy options, providing technical support to countries, and monitoring and assessing health trends.

WHO Safe Surgery Checklist — A checklist that identifies three phases of an operation, each corresponding to a specific period in the normal flow of work: Before the induction of anesthesia (sign in), before the incision of the skin (time-out), and before the patient leaves the operating room (sign out). In each phase, a checklist coordinator must confirm that the surgical team has completed the listed tasks before it proceeds with the operation.

References

AORN. (2013). *Perioperative Standards and Recommended Practices*. Denver: AORN, Inc.

AORN. (2011). *Perioperative Nursing Data Set* (3rd ed.). Denver: AORN, Inc.

Association for the Advancement of Medical Instrumentation. About AAMI. Retrieved April 2, 2013, from http://www.aami.org/about/index.html.

Centers for Disease Control and Prevention (CDC). (2011). Healthcare-associated infections (HAIs): Guidelines and recommendations. Retrieved April 2, 2013, from http://www.cdc.gov/HAI/prevent/prevent_pubs.html.

Institute for Health Improvement (IHI). (2011). World Health Organization (WHO) surgical safety checklist and getting started kit. Retrieved Feb. 5, 2013, from http://www.ihi.org/knowledge/Pages/Tools/WHOSurgicalSafetyChecklistGettingStartedKit.aspx
Note: includes a conference call recording, checklist, starter kit, and implementation manual. Registration is required to access documents, but is free and includes a weekly e-newsletter.

Odom-Forren, J. & Watson, D. (2005). *Practical Guide to Moderate Sedation/Analgesia* (2nd ed.). St. Louis: Elsevier Mosby.

Phillips, N. (2013). *Berry and Kohn's Operating Room Technique* (12th ed.). St. Louis: Mosby.

Phippen, M. L., Ulmer, B.C., & Wells, M.P. (2009). *Competency for Safe Patient Care During Operative and Invasive Procedures*. Denver: CCI.

Rothrock, J.C. (Ed.). (2011). *Alexander's Care of the Patient in Surgery* (14th ed.). St. Louis: Mosby.

World Health Organization (WHO). (2009). Surgical Safety Checklist (2nd ed.). Retrieved Feb. 5, 2013, from http://www.who.int/patientsafety/safesurgery/tools_resources/en/

Answers to Chapter 3 Activities

Module 1: Introduction of the patient to the operative/procedural area — Pages 84-87

Activity — Short Answer

Who is included in a time-out prior to surgery?
Surgeon(s), anesthesia care provider, registered nurse circulator, scrub person

Source: Phippen, M. L., Ulmer, B.C., & Wells, M.P. (2009). *Competency for Safe Patient Care During Operative and Invasive Procedures,* p. 141. Denver: CCI.

Case Study Activity

What risk factors does Mrs. M. have for developing a deep vein thrombosis?
Obesity, smoking, positioning (reverse Trendelenburg)

Sources: AORN. (2013). Recommended practices for prevention of deep vein thrombosis, pp. 366-367. In *Perioperative Standards and Recommended Practices.* Denver: AORN, Inc. Rothrock, J.C. (Ed.). (2011). *Alexander's Care of the Patient in Surgery* (14th ed., p. 162). St. Louis: Mosby.

Activity — Critical Thinking

Your patient, scheduled for a total hip arthroplasty, has stated that her religious beliefs prevent her from accepting a blood transfusion. What are your choices in fluid management that will respect her wishes?

Consider having available volume expanders (colloids and crystalloids) and an autotransfusion (cell salvage) device. Colloids (Albumin, Dextran, Hespan, etc.) and crystalloids (e.g., normal saline, lactated ringers) will assist with maintaining blood pressure but do not have oxygen carrying capabilities. Efficient use of surgical time and hemostasis will also assist in minimizing blood loss.

Source: Rothrock, J.C. (Ed.). (2011). *Alexander's Care of the Patient in Surgery* (14th ed., p. 42). St. Louis: Mosby.

Case Study Activity

1. When should Mrs. M.'s preoperative antibiotic be administered? When should it be discontinued?

Mrs. M.'s antibiotic should be administered within 60 minutes before the incision. It should be discontinued within 24 hours after surgery. Note: Due to Mrs. M.'s allergy to penicillin, her anesthesia care provider may choose not to administer cefazolin. If another antibiotic is chosen, the infusion time may vary.

Source: Rothrock, J.C. (Ed.). (2011). *Alexander's Care of the Patient in Surgery* (14th ed., p. 55). St. Louis: Mosby.

2. What should be included in Mrs. M.'s time-out?

(Sample answer)
Correct patient (identify Mrs. M.)
Correct procedure/site (laparoscopic cholecystectomy, possible open, possible cholangiograms)
Correct position (supine, reverse Trendelenburg) on radiolucent OR bed
Availability of special equipment, special requirements (supplies and equipment for an open cholecystectomy; cholangiogram supplies; extra-long instruments; notification of x-ray tech to stand by).
Suspected malignant hyperthermia
Allergies: Penicillin, suspected latex. Verify that Mrs. M. is not allergic to x-ray medium used for possible cholangiogram.
Medications: Radiopaque dye available; prophylactic antibiotic given; local anesthetic available.

Source: Phippen, M. L., Ulmer, B.C., & Wells, M.P. (2009). *Competency for Safe Patient Care During Operative and Invasive Procedures,* p. 141. Denver: CCI.

3. Mrs. M. wonders "what all the fuss is about" concerning keeping her warm. She states, "In 5 minutes, I'll be asleep, and won't even know if I'm cold or not." What do you tell her?

(Sample response; you may think of others)
Being cold is one of the most common complications of surgery. It increases the risk for getting an infection postoperatively, and may promote abnormal heart rates (ventricular tachycardia). It increases the risk for bleeding (inhibits platelet aggregation). It affects the way your body responds to medications so that it takes longer for you to wake up (alters metabolism, increases length of action of muscle relaxant). Because you're diabetic, you're at risk for being cold anyway.

Source: AORN. (2013). Recommended practices for the prevention of hypothermia, pp. 375-376. In *Perioperative Standards and Recommended Practices*. Denver: AORN, Inc.

4. From your preoperative assessment you learned that Mrs. M.'s maternal grandmother died during surgery to remove her gallbladder in 1954. Mrs. M. states "I'm really worried that the same thing is going to happen to me." How would you address Mrs. M.'s concern? What nursing interventions can you employ to decrease her anxiety?

(Sample response; yours may vary)
Concerns about dying during surgery should be taken seriously. This information should be communicated to Mrs. M.'s surgeon and anesthesiologist to follow up on a possible risk factor for malignant hyperthermia.

If Mrs. M. agrees, a hospital chaplain or her own spiritual advisor could be asked to talk with her preoperatively.

Nursing interventions to decrease your patient's anxiety include:

- *Answer questions and provide information in language that Mrs. M. can understand.*
- *Remain in close proximity to provide reassurance.*
- *Maintain a quiet environment that is focused on Mrs. M.*
- *Introduce other team members and briefly describe their roles.*
- *Provide privacy by keeping Mrs. M. covered and warm.*
- *Limit traffic in the room.*

Source: Phillips, N. (2013). *Berry and Kohn's Operating Room Technique* (12th ed., pp. 17, 102, 375, 380). St. Louis: Mosby.

5. Physiologic responses to the stress of the surgical procedure and Mrs. M.'s health assessment can trigger some unique situations for the management of her care. In reviewing her preoperative assessment, what physiologic responses might you as her intraoperative nurse encounter?

1. Mrs. M. has been NPO since midnight, yet took her regular dose of Glucophage this morning. She will need to be monitored for low blood sugars.

2. Her stated food allergies and reactions to latex products are indicative of a latex allergy. Other persons involved with her care will need to be notified, and a latex free environment initiated.

3. Obesity is a risk factor for skin breakdown. Careful attention to skin assessment, positioning and padding will need to be initiated to prevent a break in skin integrity.

4. Diagnosis of hypertension, the stress of surgery, and the emotional response to her grandmother's death during the same procedure may trigger blood pressure issues or other stress responses during the procedure. Pharmacologic and nonpharmacologic interventions will need to be implemented as required.

5. An unexplained familial death during surgery in combination with her subjective comments on exercise-induced overheating are suspicious for malignant hyperthermia (MH). The anesthesia care provider and surgeon need to be notified. Policy and resources for managing MH should be readily available for review.

Module 2: Support safe practices regarding anesthesia provider, surgeon, and nurse administered medications — Pages 88-91

Activity — Matching

1. Draw a line between the physical status classification and the corresponding patient.

P1 =   25-year-old male, healthy, taking no medications
P2 =   48-year-old male, diabetes mellitus Type II, takes Glyburide. Hemoglobin A1c is 6.9
P3 =   64-year-old female, history of hypertension; typically runs 150/90 to 165/100 mmHg with medication
P4 =   72-year-old male, diabetes mellitus Type II, COPD, on dialysis and oxygen 2L/min nasal cannula
P5 =   86-year-old female, multisystem trauma from head-on motor vehicle accident

2. Circle the patients appropriate for nurse-monitored moderate sedation.

Circle patients P1 and P2 (P3 is not medically stable).

Source: AORN. (2013). Recommended practices for managing the patient receiving moderate sedation/analgesia, p. 416. In *Perioperative Standards and Recommended Practices.* Denver: AORN.

Activity — Critical Thinking

1. You are caring for an 18-month-old patient undergoing bilateral myringotomy with insertion of ear tubes. The surgeon asks you to give an acetaminophen (Tylenol) suppository. The child weighs 26 pounds. The dose is 10 mg/kg, and the drug is supplied in 80, 120, and 325 mg suppositories.

A. What is the correct route and dosage for this drug for this patient?

Rectal; 26 pounds = 11.8 kg X 10 mg = 118 mg of drug needed.
Administer the 120 mg suppository.

B. What else will you need to do to correctly administer this drug?

Confirm patient identity and presence of any allergies or contraindications. Confirm weight-based dosing and "read back" the order before administration. Use hand hygiene before and after administration of the suppository. Wear a non-sterile glove, and moisten the end of the suppository to ease insertion. Document order and drug, dose, route, and time given in patient record.

Source: AORN. (2013). Recommended practices for medication safety, pp. 263, 265-266, 269-270. In *Perioperative Standards and Recommended Practices.* Denver: AORN, Inc.

2. You work in a cardiac cath lab and frequently monitor patients undergoing moderate sedation/anesthesia. What monitoring equipment should be provided for safe patient care?

The recommended equipment for monitoring a patient undergoing moderate sedation is the same regardless of setting. Blood pressure, EKG, and oxygen saturation monitors should be used for every patient. Respiratory rate, pulse rate and rhythm, blood pressure, oxygen saturation, level of consciousness, and skin condition should be monitored at least every 15 minutes throughout the procedure, and after administration of every medication.

Source: Rothrock, J.C. (Ed.). (2011). *Alexander's Care of the Patient in Surgery* (14th ed., p. 137). St. Louis: Mosby.

Activity — Do You Know?

You are monitoring a patient undergoing a central venous catheter insertion under moderate sedation. The surgeon asks you to give an initial dose of 3 mg of midazolam (Versed) IV push. You would (circle the correct response):

A. Question the surgeon. The amount is lower than the normal range for the initial recommended dose.
B. Question the surgeon. The amount is higher than the normal range for the initial recommended dose.
C. Give the dose. It is within the normal range for the initial recommended dose.

B. The normal range for the initial dose for this drug is 1.5-2 mg. The initial titrated dose should not exceed 2.5 mg.

Source: Odom-Forren, J. & Watson, D. (2005). *Practical Guide to Moderate Sedation/Analgesia* (2nd ed., p. 62). St. Louis: Elsevier Mosby.

Case Study Activity

Based on Mrs. M.'s history, which anesthetic(s) should be avoided?

Halothane, Isoflurane, Enflurane, Sevoflurane, Desflurane, and Succinylcholine

Source: Malignant Hyperthermia Association of the United States (MHAUS). (2011). *Anesthetics*. Retrieved Feb. 5, 2013, from http://www.mhaus.org/anesthetics/.

Activity — Short Answer

1.You are caring for a patient scheduled for a laparoscopic Nissen fundoplication. When you arrive to interview the patient, you find him sitting up at a 45-degree angle. He states that when he lies flat, he "gets terrible heartburn." What is the risk for this patient in undergoing a general anesthetic? What can you anticipate your anesthesiologist will need?

This patient is at risk for aspiration due to his diagnosis of hiatal hernia and history of esophageal reflux. You can anticipate that your anesthesiologist will perform a rapid sequence induction. You should have the difficult airway equipment available and be prepared to provide cricoid (Sellick maneuver) pressure.

Source: Rothrock, J.C. (Ed.). (2011). *Alexander's Care of the Patient in Surgery* (14th ed., p. 129). St. Louis: Mosby.

Module 3: Incorporate principles of safe positioning — Pages 91-94

Activity — X Marks the Spot

Mark with an "X" the corresponding pressure points associated with the following patient positions. *(See figures on next page.)*

Sources: Rothrock, J.C. (Ed.). (2011). *Alexander's Care of the Patient in Surgery* (14th ed., pp. 162-163). St. Louis: Mosby. Phillips, N. (2013). *Berry and Kohn's Operating Room Technique* (12th ed., pp. 493, 502-508). St. Louis: Mosby. Phippen, M. L., Ulmer, B.C., & Wells, M.P. (2009). *Competency for Safe Patient Care During Operative and Invasive Procedures*, pp. 192-209. Denver: CCI.

Supine

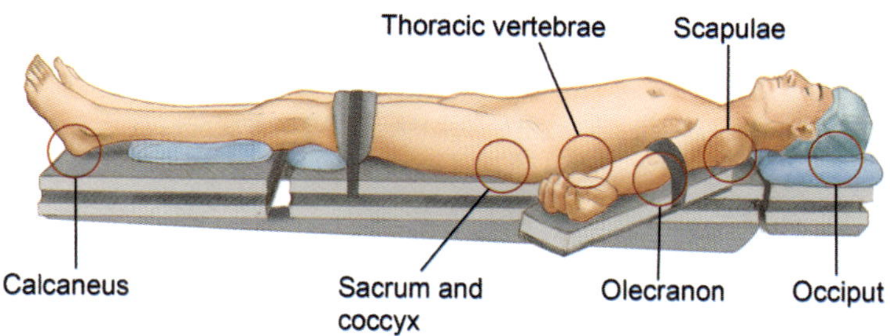

Prone

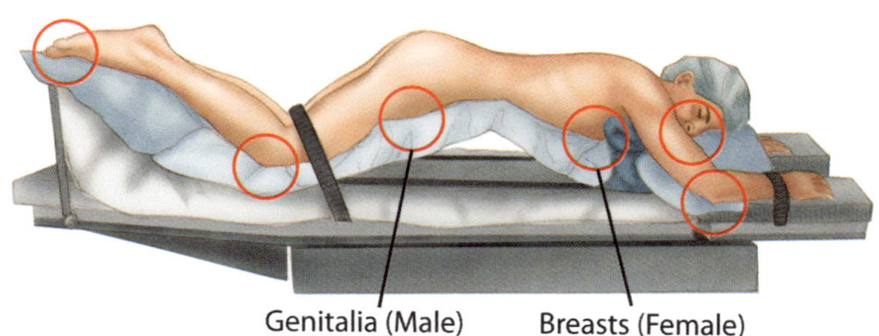

Lithotomy, boot stirrups

Sitting

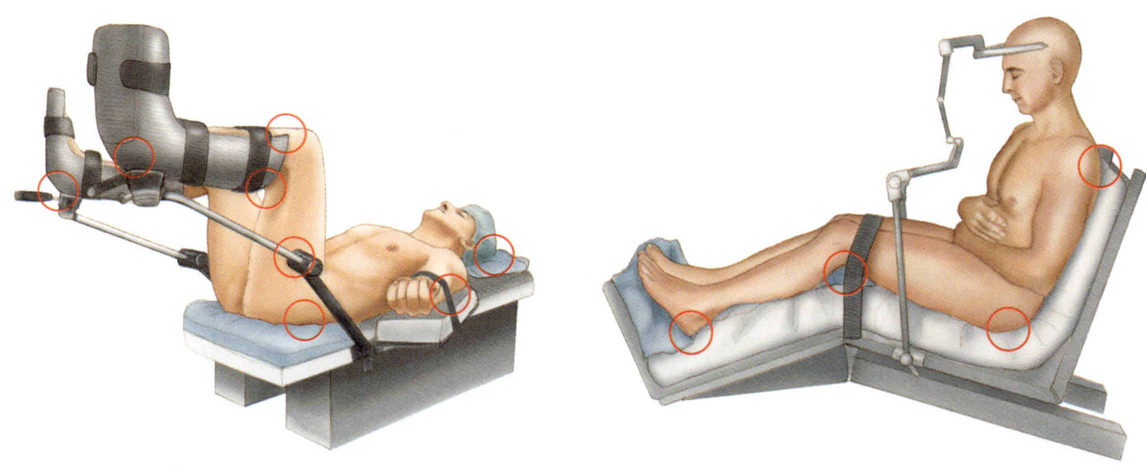

Lateral decubitis

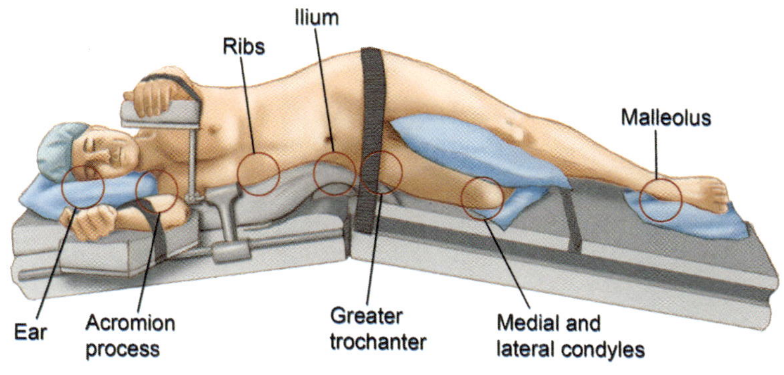

Activity — Circle the Correct Answer

In the left lateral decubitis position, the patient is lying on the *LEFT* side.

Source: Phippen, M. L., Ulmer, B.C., & Wells, M.P. (2009). *Competency for Safe Patient Care During Operative and Invasive Procedures,* pp. 192-209. Denver: CCI.

Activity — Matching

Match the position with the associated nerve injury. Answers may be used more than once.

Supine - *A, E*	A. brachial plexus
Lithotomy - *B, C*	B.peroneal
Lateral - *A, B*	C. saphenous
Prone - *A, E, F*	D. sciatic
Semi-Fowler - *A*	E. ulnar
Fowler - *E*	F. radial

Source: Rothrock, J.C. (Ed.). (2011). *Alexander's Care of the Patient in Surgery* (14th ed., pp. 162-173). St. Louis: Mosby.

Activity — Do You Know?

The preferred placement for the patient's arms in the prone position are *at the patient's sides.*

Source: AORN. (2013). Recommended practices for positioning the patient, p. 433. In *Perioperative Standards and Recommended Practices.* Denver: AORN, Inc.

Module 4: Prepare the surgical site — Pages 94-99

Activity — Critical Thinking

You are caring for a patient who is scheduled for reanastomosis of a colostomy. How is the typical skin prep adjusted for this patient?

Surgical preps should normally start at the incision site and move to the periphery. If the incision site is more highly contaminated (e.g., the colostomy) than the surrounding skin, the area with a lower bacterial count should be prepped first. An antiseptic-soaked sponge may be applied to the contaminated area during the prep of the surrounding skin.

Source: AORN. (2013). Recommended practices for preoperative patient skin antisepsis, p. 82. In *Perioperative Standards and Recommended Practices.* Denver: AORN, Inc.

Activity — Color Me

For each illustration, mark the incision (if applicable) and shade the area to be prepped.
See figures below and on following pages.

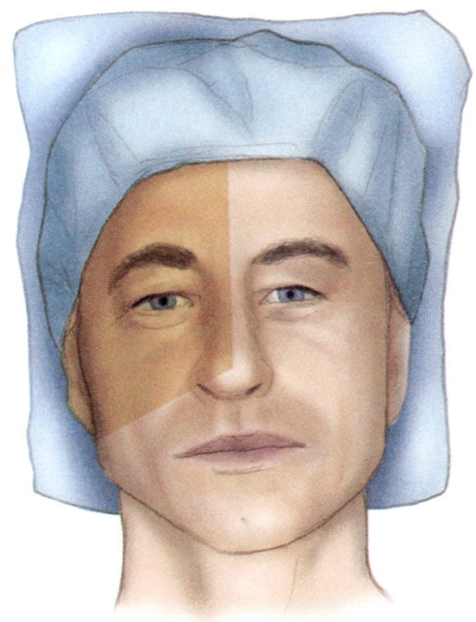

Cataract extraction, right eye

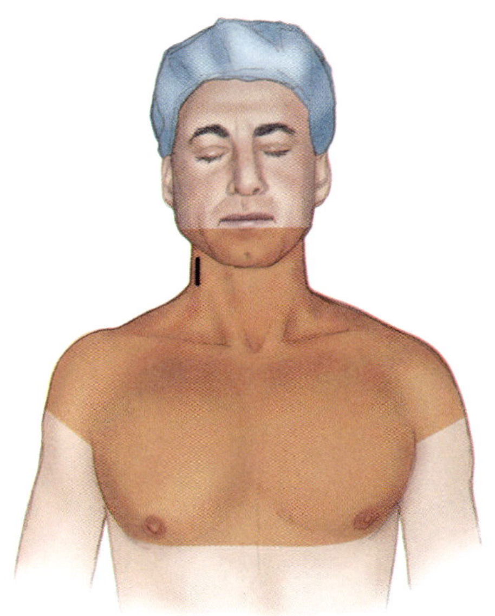

Right carotid endarterectomy

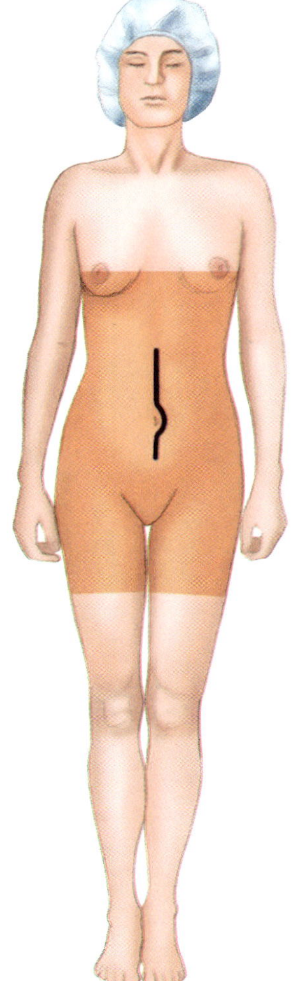

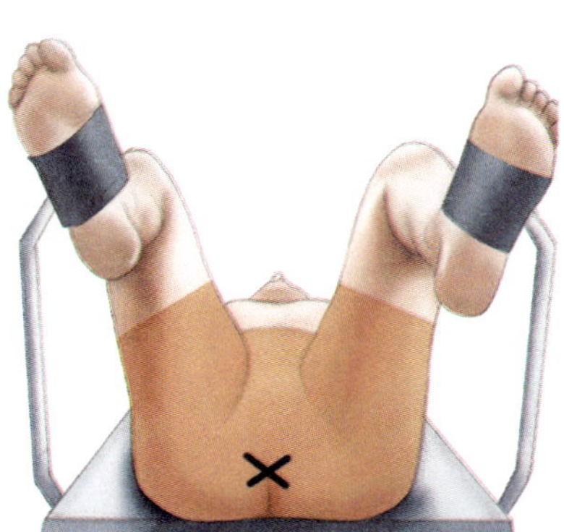

Abdominal/perineal resection

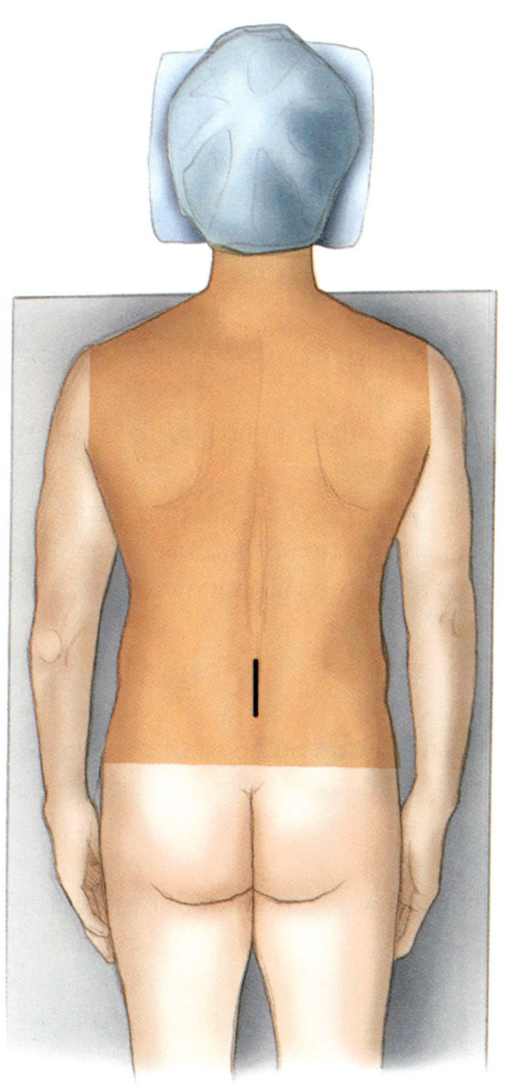

Lumbar discectomy, L4-L5

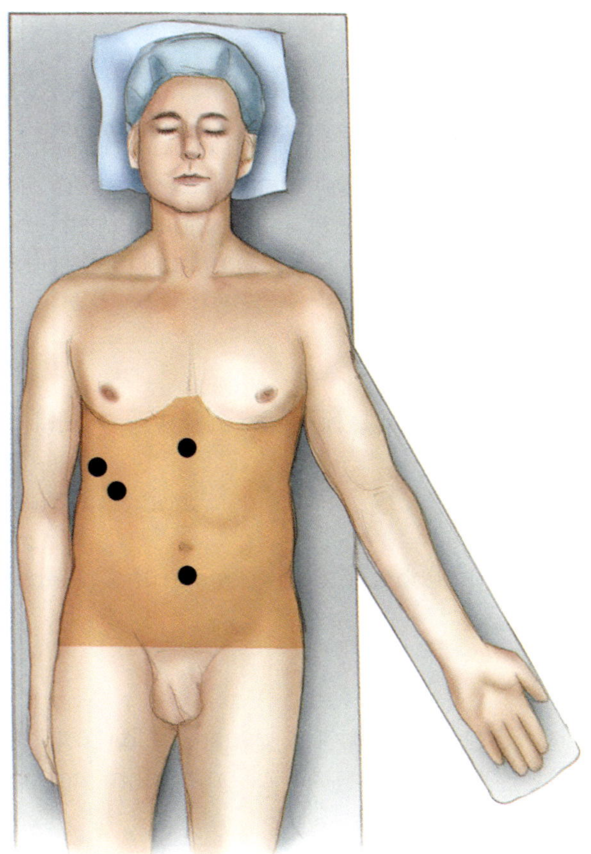

Laparoscopic cholecystectomy

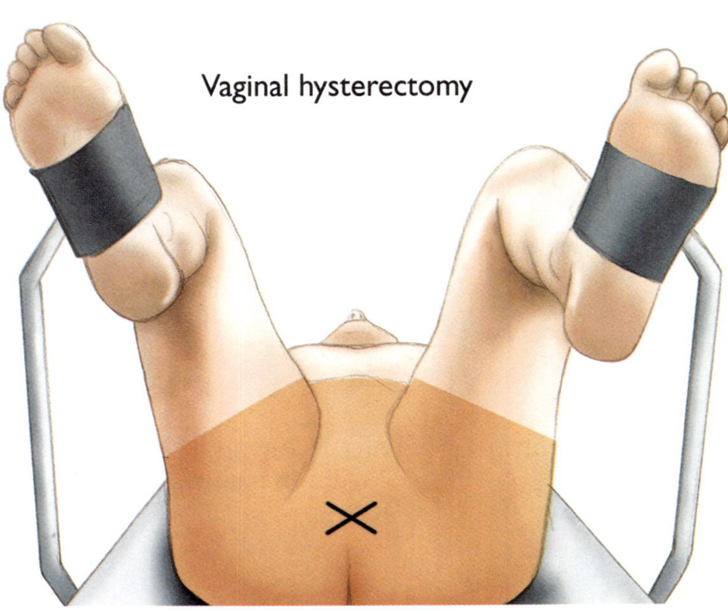

Vaginal hysterectomy

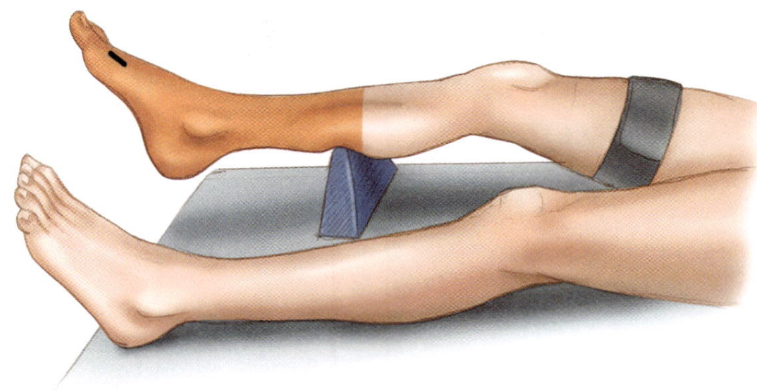

Right bunionectomy

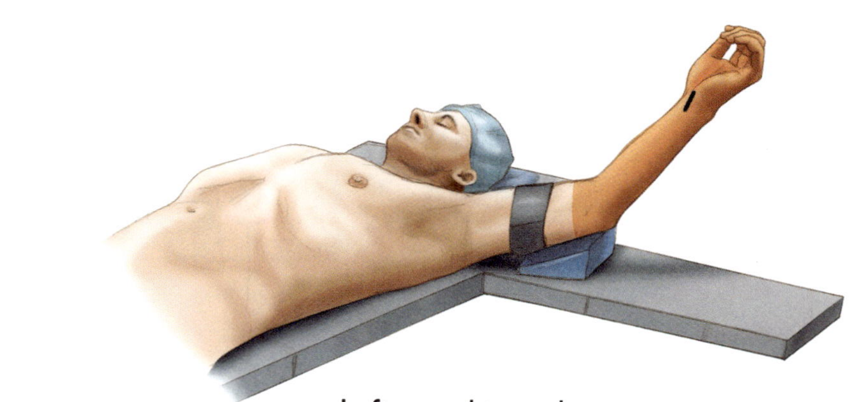

Left carpal tunnel

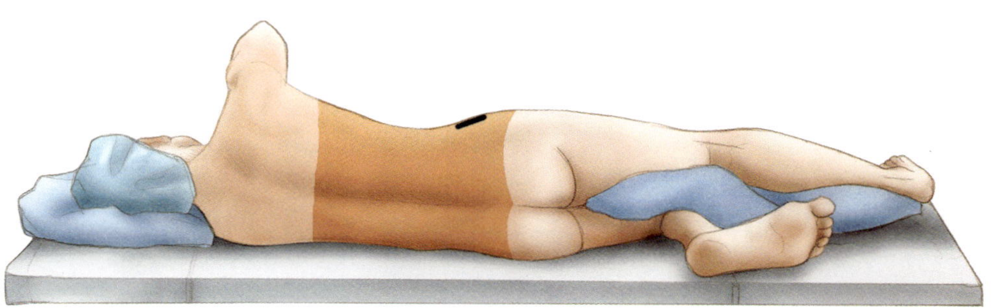

Right nephrectomy

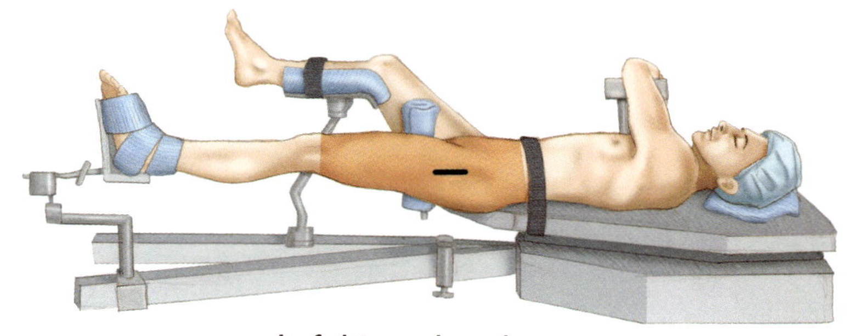

Left hip arthroplasty

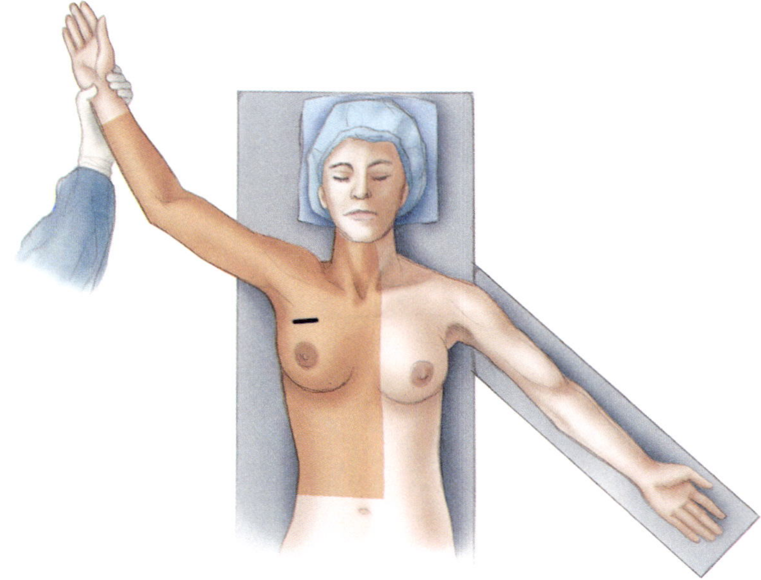

Source: Phippen, M. L., Ulmer, B.C., & Wells, M.P. (2009). *Competency for Safe Patient Care During Operative and Invasive Procedures*, pp. 258-265. Denver: CCI.

Right lumpectomy, right upper quadrant

Activity — Critical Thinking

The surgeon requests that hair be removed from the immediate incisional area for an extremely hirsute male scheduled for an inguinal herniorraphy. What is the best method for accomplishing this?

If hair must be removed, it is recommended to be done the day of surgery, in a location outside the OR, with a clipper that is either single-use or with a reusable head that can be disinfected between patients. Only hair that is directly interfering with the surgical procedure should be removed. A razor should not be used as it increases the risk of surgical site infection. A depilatory may be used, but carries with it the increased risk for hypersensitivity reactions.

Source: AORN. (2013). Recommended practices for preoperative patient skin antisepsis, p. 80. In *Perioperative Standards and Recommended Practices*. Denver: AORN, Inc.

Module 5: Apply principles of asepsis — Pages 100-102

Activity — Matching

Match the area with the required appropriate attire. Answers may be used more than once.

Cafeteria: ***E***

Sterile supply room: ***B, C, D***

OR with opened supplies: ***A, B, C, D***

A. mask
B. surgical scrubs
C. hair covering
D. coverall/jumpsuit
E. street clothes

Source: AORN. (2013). Recommended practices for traffic patterns, p. 121. In *Perioperative Standards and Recommended Practices*. Denver: AORN, Inc.

Activity — Fill In the Blank

For the following procedures, write in the corresponding wound classification:

Total knee replacement: ***Clean wound, Class I***

Incision and drainage of abscess, status postop posterior spinal fusion: ***Dirty/infected wound, Class IV***

Appendectomy, unruptured: ***Clean/Contaminated wound, Class II***

Open reduction internal fixation open fracture right radius/ulna: ***Contaminated wound, Class III***

Source: Rothrock, J.C. (Ed.). (2011). *Alexander's Care of the Patient in Surgery* (14th ed., pp. 254, 256). St. Louis: Mosby.

Activity — Short Answer

1. You are turning over your room for a cystoscopy for a 7-year-old girl. You drop an unopened box of 4X4 radiopaque sponges on the floor. What should you do?

The box and its contents should be discarded. The paper lid is not impervious, and moisture from the freshly mopped floor could have contaminated the contents.

Source: Rothrock, J.C. (Ed.). (2011). *Alexander's Care of the Patient in Surgery* (14th ed., p. 86). St. Louis: Mosby

2. You are scrubbed for a lumpectomy for a 44-year-old woman. The surgeon asks you to move to the other side of the table to hold a retractor. What is the appropriate way to pass the other scrubbed members of the team?

Members should pass face-to-face or back-to-back while maintaining safe distances from the sterile field.

Source: AORN. (2013). Recommended practices for maintaining a sterile field, p. 110. In *Perioperative Standards and Recommended Practices*. Denver: AORN, Inc.

Module 6: Provide perioperative nursing care during operative and invasive procedures — Pages 102-105

"Go To" Case Study Activity

From your previously developed concept map and the patient assessment, develop a plan of care for the intraoperative component of Mrs. M.'s perioperative experience.

1. Identify the nursing interventions that will need to be used for Mrs. M.'s surgical procedure. Some of these are typical for every surgery (e.g., infection prevention, principles of aseptic technique, skin antisepsis), while others will be specific for Mrs. M. ***(See CD for sample answers.)***

2. Arrange the intraoperative activities from your list under their corresponding "major problems" boxes you developed in Chapters 1 and 2. *(See CD for sample answers.)*

3. What critical information needs to be communicated to the following health care team members?

Anesthesia provider: ***Low potassium, possible latex allergy, risk factor for malignant hyperthermia, status of current medications***

Surgeon: ***Low potassium, possible latex allergy, risk factor for malignant hyperthermia, status of current medications***

Scrub person: ***Possible latex allergy, risk factor for malignant hyperthermia***

PACU: ***Low potassium, possible latex allergy, risk factor for malignant hyperthermia, status of current medications, intraoperative blood glucose results***

Activity — Short Answer

A 17-year-old patient returns to your facility seven months postoperatively for removal of an infected Harrington rod implant. The wound cultures *Staphylococcus aureus*. Is this considered a surgical site infection? Why or why not?

Yes. This is considered a surgical site infection. The infection occurred within one year of insertion of the implant and was confirmed with an aseptically obtained culture.

Source: Rothrock, J.C. (Ed.). (2011). *Alexander's Care of the Patient in Surgery* (14th ed., p. 254). St. Louis: Mosby.

Activity — Name That Incision

Name the abdominal incisions in the diagram.

Source: Rothrock, J.C. (Ed.). (2011). *Alexander's Care of the Patient in Surgery* (14th ed., p. 312). St. Louis: Mosby.

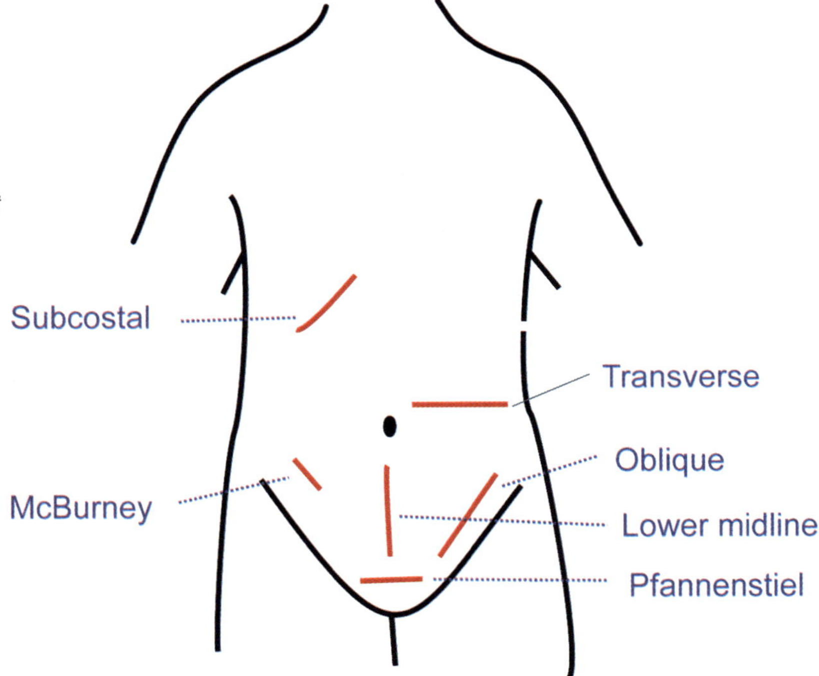

Activity — Matching

Match the incision types shown in the illustration on page 134 to their corresponding surgical procedure. Use each answer only once.

Lower midline: *C*
Oblique: *D*
Pfannenstiel: *A*
Subcostal: *E*
McBurney: *B*
Transverse: *F*

A. abdominal hysterectomy
B. appendectomy
C. radical retropubic prostatectomy
D. open inguinal herniorraphy
E. hepatic resection
F. choledochojejunostomy

Source: Rothrock, J.C. (Ed.). (2011). *Alexander's Care of the Patient in Surgery* (14th ed., pp. 312-315, 527). St. Louis: Mosby.

Activity — Short Answer

Your patient is scheduled for an ulnar nerve release, left elbow; he states that he has an implantable cardiodefibrillator. What is the safest electrosurgical method to use, and why?

The bipolar ESU provides hemostasis at the surgical site with less potential stimulation of adjacent tissue. Because the active and return electrodes are contained in the tips of the instrument, the current passes between the two poles and only affects the tissue between the poles. There is less chance of stray or alternate pathways with this form of electrocautery. Bipolar electrosurgery uses a lower voltage so that there is less potential for electromagnetic interference.

Sources: AORN. (2013). Recommended practices for electrosurgery, pp. 126, 133. In *Perioperative Standards and Recommended Practices*. Denver: AORN, Inc.; Phippen, M. L., Ulmer, B.C., & Wells, M.P. (2009). *Competency for Safe Patient Care During Operative and Invasive Procedures,* p. 512. Denver: CCI.

Module 7: Identify and control environmental factors — Pages 105-108

Activity — Fill in the Blank

For each of the following environmental control, list the acceptable parameters:

Air exchanges:
OR: *minimum 15/hour, recommended 20-25;* Cardiac cath lab: *15/hour;* Sterile storage area: *4/hour;* Decontamination area: *at least 6/hour*

Humidity:
OR: *30-60%;* Cardiac cath lab: *30-60%;* Decontamination area: *30-60%*

Temperature:
OR: *68°F-73°F;* Cardiac cath lab: *70°F-75°F;* Decontamination area: *68°F-73°F*

Air pressure in the OR should be *greater* than the surrounding corridors.

Source: AORN. (2013). Recommended practices for: Minimally invasive surgery, p. 161; Cleaning and care of instruments and powered equipment, p. 489; Sterilization, p. 529. In *Perioperative Standards and Recommended Practices*. Denver: AORN, Inc; Rothrock, J.C. (Ed.). (2011). *Alexander's Care of the Patient in Surgery* (14th ed., p. 67). St. Louis: Mosby.

Activity — Short Answer

For each source of noise, list a nursing intervention to reduce its risk of disrupting the environment and impacting patient safety:

Examples of interventions include the following (you may think of others).

Beeper/pager/cell phone: *Place on silent whenever possible.*

Monitor alarms: *Turn to the lowest setting that is still audible.*

Electronic music devices (radios, CD players): *Turn to the lowest setting that is still audible. Requests to turn off distracting music should be honored.*

Overhead pages and announcements: *Use text paging.*

Telephones: *Limit conversations to brief communication. Practice telephone etiquette when answering the phone.*

Staff communication:
Minimize the number of people present during procedures and limit traffic flow.
Establish and enforce times when noise levels should be routinely be reduced (e.g., induction, emergence, counts).
Use a low speaking voice, and remind others to do the same.
Increase staff awareness via education.
Post signs to remind staff to keep noise levels low.
Minimize irrelevant conversation.

Sources: Rothrock, J.C. (Ed.). (2011). *Alexander's Care of the Patient in Surgery* (14th ed., p. 113). St. Louis: Mosby; AORN. (2009). Position statement on noise in the perioperative setting. Retrieved Feb. 6, 2013, from http://www.aorn.org/Clinical_Practice/Position_Statements/Position_Statements.aspx

Case Study Activity

As the anesthesia care provider hands you a tube of blood for a blood chemistry analysis for Mrs. M., it slips out of your hand and drops to the floor, breaking the tube. What is the best way to clean up the spill?

Gloves must be worn; the broken tube should be placed in the sharps container. The blood should be removed with a lint-free cloth, and the area disinfected with an EPA-registered disinfectant as soon as possible. The contaminated cleaning cloth should be placed in a designated biohazardous receptacle. The gloves used during cleaning the spill should be removed, and hand hygiene performed.

in the room before activating the equipment. All staff should wear protective shielding (aprons, thyroid shields). Preoperative assessment should include verifying any allergies or contraindications to x-ray medium.

Source: AORN. (2013). Recommended practices for reducing radiological exposure, pp. 296-298. In *Perioperative Standards and Recommended Practices*. Denver: AORN, Inc.

3. Dr. S. repeatedly asks for the coagulation power on the electrosurgical unit to be increased. You know that a need for abnormally high settings may indicate a problem with the system. What steps should be taken in trouble-shooting a possible problem?

- *Confirm power settings with surgeon; communicate what "normal" settings are based on manufacturer's recommendations.*
- *Check patient return electrode to make certain it is in good contact with the patient.*
- *Check all connections (patient return electrode, electrode cord, and power cord) to ensure that they are plugged in correctly.*
- *Check for presence of an alternate ground (EKG electrode, Mrs. M.'s body in contact with metal).*
- *Replace patient return electrode if necessary; if problem continues, remove electrosurgical unit from service. Send patient return electrode and unit to the biomedical department for evaluation.*
- *Carefully assess Mrs. M. for undetected thermal injuries.*

Sources: AORN. (2013). Recommended practices for electrosurgery, pp. 126-127. In *Perioperative Standards and Recommended Practices*. Denver: AORN, Inc.; Phippen, M. L., Ulmer, B.C., & Wells, M.P. (2009). *Competency for Safe Patient Care During Operative and Invasive Procedures,* p. 314. Denver: CCI.

4. Upon completion of the surgery, a slightly reddened area is noted on Mrs. M.'s left thigh under the electrosurgical dispersive electrode. As her nurse, what steps do you need to take to document this incident?

Sample responses; yours may vary:
Note that the variance report example below contains more specific details than the patient record. The fact that an occurrence/variance form was completed should NOT be documented in the patient's permanent record.

- *Patient record: "Patient dispersive electrode removed at end of procedure. Reddened area noted under electrode approximately 2 inches by 3 inches at the distal end of dispersive electrode site. Dr. Smith notified. Silvadene cream applied per his order."*
- *Variance report: "Patient dispersive electrode removed at end of procedure. Reddened area noted under pad area approximately 2 inches by 3 inches at the distal end of dispersive electrode site. Dr. Smith notified. Electrosurgery unit #5 removed from service and sent to biomedical department for evaluation, along with grounding pad, serial number 453S2. All other grounding pads with same serial number removed from stock and quarantined."*

Source: Phillips, N. (2013). *Berry and Kohn's Operating Room Technique* (12th ed., p. 50). St. Louis: Mosby.

Module 9: Prepare and label specimens — Pages 112-113

Activity — Short Answer

Identification of the specimen should be confirmed verbally between the circulating nurse and the surgeon using a "read back" communication similar to that used with verbal orders. What information needs to be communicated between the surgeon and circulating nurse?

Originating source of specimen (e.g., right or left, site)
Type of tissue
Clinical diagnosis
Any pertinent information (e.g., patient history, suture marking for orientation, requests for tests)

Source: AORN. (2013). Recommended practices for specimen care and handling, pp. 323-324. In *Perioperative Standards and Recommended Practices*. Denver: AORN, Inc.

Activity — True or False

1. Formalin is considered a hazardous chemical that should be disposed of according to OSHA regulations.
   False; formalin disposal is regulated by the Environmental Protection Agency.

2. The specimen label should be placed on the lid of the container.
   False; the label should be placed on the container.

Source: AORN. (2013). Recommended practices for specimen care and handling, pp. 324-325. In *Perioperative Standards and Recommended Practices*. Denver: AORN, Inc.

Module 10: Perform counts — Pages 113-115

Activity — Do You Know?

How many strategies can you list to help prevent a retained surgical item?

Sample responses:
Avoid unnecessary distractions/talking, which interfere with clear communication between circulator and scrub person.
Immediately document items added to the count.
Account for counted items that have fallen/been removed from the sterile field.
Perform counts consistently in a standardized manner to minimize chance for error.
Keep sterile field organized.
Confine sharps to a designated area.
Use only radiopaque items in the wound.
Report discrepancies in count immediately.
Verify items concurrently.

Source: AORN. (2013). Recommended practices for prevention of retained surgical items, pp. 306-309. In *Perioperative Standards and Recommended Practices*. Denver: AORN, Inc.

Activity — Critical Thinking

You are counting sponges with the scrub person in preparation for an abdominal hysterectomy. The package of 4X4 radiopaque sponges you have opened contains 9 sponges instead of 10. What should you do?

Packages containing an incorrect number of radiopaque sponges should be removed from the room before the patient arrives to decrease confusion and minimize the likelihood for error.

Source: AORN. (2013). Recommended practices for prevention of retained surgical items, p. 308. In *Perioperative Standards and Recommended Practices*. Denver: AORN, Inc.

Activity — Scramble

Number the following steps in the correct order for completing a sponge and suture count.

1. Before the procedure
2. Before closure of a cavity (e.g., uterus or bladder) within a cavity
3. When wound (peritoneum) closure begins
4. At skin closure

List two other circumstances when a count should be performed:

1. Whenever new items are added
2. At the time of permanent relief of either scrub person or circulator

Source: AORN. (2013). Recommended practices for prevention of retained surgical items, pp. 308, 310. In *Perioperative Standards and Recommended Practices*. Denver: AORN, Inc.

Case Study Activity

Mrs. M.'s surgery is near completion. As a needle holder and needle were returned to the scrub person, he noted that the needle was bent with the tip of the needle missing. Explain your immediate course of action to prevent a retained surgical item. How would you document these issues and the patient care you provided?

The circulator must notify the surgeon immediately of the missing piece of needle so that the surgeon can do a methodical wound search to look for the item. The sterile field, Mayo stand, back table, floor, kick bucket, and discarded items must be searched. If the item is found and retrieved, then the count can be documented as correct. If the surgeon and scrub nurse cannot find the needle tip, then an x-ray must be ordered. The x-ray should be read by a radiologist and a report sent to the operating room. If the needle tip is not recovered, then the count must be documented as incorrect, the results of the x-ray must be documented, and an occurrence or variance report must be completed.

Sources: AORN. (2013). Recommended practices for prevention of retained surgical items, pp. 310-311, 313-314. In *Perioperative Standards and Recommended Practices*. Denver: AORN, Inc.; AORN. (2011). *Perioperative Nursing Data Set* (PNDS). (3rd. ed., pp. 146-149).

Denver: AORN, Inc.; Phippen, M. L., Ulmer, B.C., & Wells, M.P. (2009). *Competency for Safe Patient Care During Operative and Invasive Procedures,* pp. 287-289. Denver: CCI; Rothrock, J.C. (Ed.). (2011). *Alexander's Care of the Patient in Surgery* (14th ed., p. 189). St. Louis: Mosby.

Module 11: Maintain accurate patient records — Pages 116-117

Activity — Critical Thinking

You work in a free-standing ambulatory surgery center that enjoys a thriving plastic surgery practice. Your facility has just received a letter from the FDA recalling a certain brand of breast implant. What information from the patients' records do you need to have in determining which of your patients are affected by this recall?

Name and contact information of patient
Name and contact information of the surgeon
Name of manufacturer/distributor
Lot, model, and serial numbers
Type and size of implant
Expiration date as appropriate
Any other information as requested by the FDA

Sources: Rothrock, J.C. (Ed.). (2011). *Alexander's Care of the Patient in Surgery* (14th ed., p. 893). St. Louis: Mosby.

CHAPTER 4:
Communication

Test Specifications:
9% of CNOR test questions are based on Communication.

Introduction

Have you ever gone past a piece of equipment in the hall with a sign taped to it that says "Broken"? Although this information is useful in determining that it shouldn't be used, there is no guidance related to who is responsible for repairs or the exact nature of the problem. Extra time and effort is expended to track down and recover the information needed to actually get the equipment repaired and back in service. If the information obtained is inaccurate or incomplete, there's a good chance that the repair may not be done correctly, if at all.

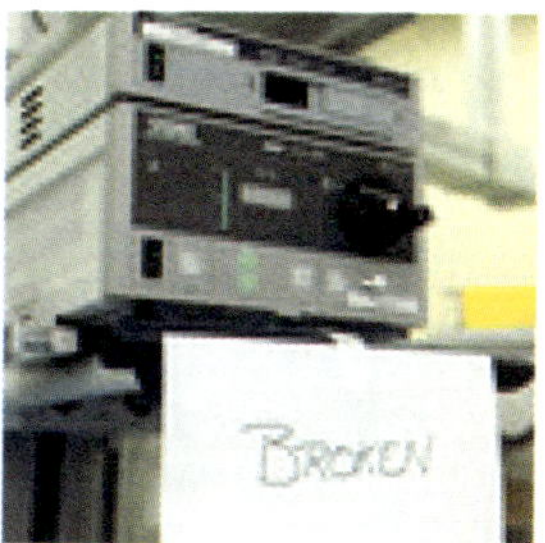

Miscommunication is not limited to equipment repairs. The Joint Commission (2009) found that communication errors were found in approximately 30% of the surgical exchanges studied; one third resulted in actions that jeopardized patient safety.

Perioperative patient care is delivered by a multidisciplinary team of health care practitioners, with no single member of the team having the knowledge to develop a comprehensive plan of care without input from other members of the team. It is through communication that we access knowledge about our patients and interact with our colleagues. Each person who interacts with the patient gathers information to support his or her clinical perspective.

This chapter will help you to apply communication strategies to a variety of learning activities. Clinical scenarios and case studies provide opportunities to identify, prioritize, and transmit information that will promote safe patient care.

Module 1: Verbal and Nonverbal Communication

Delivering the best care possible requires the perioperative nurse to solicit input from others and to communicate consistently, clearly, and assertively. Although the basic concepts of communication are the same, listening is especially important in a hectic environment such as the OR. The perioperative setting is unique in that decisions are often communicated quickly, under stressful and noisy conditions, with limited facial visual clues, and with serious ramifications if an error is made in either the transmission or receipt of the message.

Safe nursing care depends on nurses who can communicate effectively. "Reading back" has been found to be a useful way to verify what has been heard (e.g., "lobe" vs. "node" when receiving a specimen from the field).

Competency Outcomes

To successfully complete the activities in this module, you will need to be able to:

1. Identify effective communication strategies to promote quality patient outcomes.
2. Implement standardized communication processes.

Recommended Readings

Alexander's Care of the Patient in Surgery. (2011, 14th ed.), Chapter 1: Concepts basic to perioperative nursing; Chapter 2: Patient safety and risk management.

Perioperative Standards and Recommended Practices. (2013),
• Recommended practices: Transfer of patient care information.

AORN. (2011). Position statement: Creating a practice environment of safety. Retrieved Feb. 21, 2013, from http://www.aorn.org/Clinical_Practice/Position_Statements/Position_Statements.aspx

Berry and Kohn's Operating Room Technique. (2013, 12th ed.), Chapter 6: Administration of perioperative patient care services; Chapter 7: The patient: The reason for your existence; Chapter 21: Preoperative preparation of the patient.

Key Words

Communication, culture of safety, handoff, read back, SBAR, standardized communication plan, Universal Protocol, WHO checklist

Activity — Short Answer

Closed-ended (directive) questions are answered using "yes" or "no." An open-ended or non-directive question offers an opportunity to expand on the answer.

For each closed-ended (directive) preoperative interview question listed below, provide an associated open-ended (non-directive) question. Compare the differences in quality and quantity of information received utilizing both approaches.

1. Have you had anything to eat or drink in the past eight hours?

2. Is your name John?

3. Are you undergoing an appendectomy today?

4. Do you need any other help today?

Case Study Activity

1. What part of Mrs. M.'s assessment requires an immediate intervention?

2. Use the SBAR (Situation, Background, Assessment, Recommendation) format to describe how you would communicate this information to the surgeon and anesthesia care provider.

Activity — Critical Thinking

A 38-year-old female was admitted to the OR for a scheduled left L3-L4 decompression laminectomy. The consent was confirmed, and correct side and level were verified verbally and marked with the patient's participation in the preoperative area by the preoperative nurse. X-ray images were with the patient and placed on the viewer in the assigned OR. The OR was set up for a left-sided laminectomy with the electrosurgery unit (ESU) and bipolar cautery pedals placed on the floor according to the physician's preference card for a left-sided laminectomy. The patient was anesthetized, intubated, placed in the prone position, prepped, and draped by the surgical assistant before the surgeon's arrival in the OR.

The surgeon reviewed the x-rays on the viewer, and abruptly requested that the nurse move the ESU and bipolar cautery pedals to the other side. The nurse did not question his request for the change or re-verify the x-rays, but repositioned the pedals accordingly. The nurse was out of the room retrieving sutures during the time-out, but the surgeon verified the site and side with the anesthesiologist, and the surgery began on time.

The circulating nurse documented that the time-out had occurred and that all components of the Universal Protocol had been met after verifying the information directly with the anesthesiologist.

At the conclusion of the procedure, the physician reviewed the postoperative x-rays, history and physical exam findings, and consent forms only to realize he had operated on the wrong side. The patient was taken to recovery, where she was informed of the wrong-side surgery. She was returned to the OR for a second procedure.

1. Highlight the areas in the scenario above in which breaks in communication or protocol influenced patient outcomes. Then compare those areas with the analysis of the discussion in the answer section.

2. What should be done to prevent the above situation from reoccurring?

Activity — Critical Thinking

As she leaves the room to get additional suture, the circulating nurse asks the student she is precepting to put sterile saline in the basin opened on the ring stand. When she returns, she sees an unopened bottle of sterile saline sitting in the basin. How could this situation have been avoided?

<table>
<tr>
<td>

"Go To" Activity — Check It Out!

Go to Question #13, Healthy Work environment, under the Perioperative question of the week tab on your CD for an additional critical-thinking activity related to communication in the workplace.

</td>
<td>

"Go To" Activity — Skill Building

Review the Universal Protocol and WHO checklists. How do they differ? How does your facility's perioperative safety checklist compare with these two documents?

</td>
</tr>
</table>

Additional Readings

Agency for Healthcare Research and Quality. (n.d.). Never Events. Retrieved Feb. 21, 2013, from http://psnet.ahrq.gov/primer.aspx?primerID=3

AORN. (2012). Patient hand-off toolkit. Retrieved Feb. 21, 2013, from http://www.aorn.org/Secondary.aspx?id=20849

AORN, Vitalsmarts, & AACN. The Silent Treatment: Why safety tools and checklists aren't enough to save lives. Retrieved Feb. 21, 2013, from http://silenttreatmentstudy.com/

Gawande, A. (2010). *The checklist manifesto.* New York, NY: Henry Holt and Co.

The Joint Commision. (2013). National Patient Safety Goals. Retrieved Feb. 21, 2013, from http://www.jointcommission.org/standards_information/npsgs.aspx

Watson, D.S. (2009). Implementing the Universal Protocol. *AORN Journal, 90*(2), 283-287.

World Health Organization (WHO). (2009). *Safe surgery saves lives.* Retrieved Feb. 21, 2013, from http://www.who.int/patientsafety/safesurgery/en/

Module 2: Written Communication

Written documentation, either a physical chart or an electronic record, should provide consistent, accessible information, and as such is a prime communication tool for managing patient care safely and effectively among multidisciplinary health care providers. Documentation must be clear, concise, objective, and complete, because multidisciplinary caregivers rely heavily on written communication in making patient care decisions.

Nurses learn very early that "if it wasn't documented, it wasn't done!" Observations and patient interventions that are not documented are unavailable to other team members to help with decision making related to patient care. Because accurate information is integral to planning appropriate patient care, failing to document, documenting poorly, or documenting incorrectly are all serious errors with a significant impact on patient outcomes.

Remember — the chart is a legal document. Unexpected events often trigger an investigation, and it will be very difficult for you to remember the details months or years afterward. Having comprehensive documentation of the facts is essential for performance improvement audits, perioperative nursing research, and risk mitigation.

Competency Outcomes

To successfully complete the activities in this module, you will need to be able to:

1. Describe best practices in written communication that promote quality patient care outcomes.
2. Identify regulatory influences on written communication in the health care setting.
3. Discuss the legal implications of written documentation.

Recommended Reading

Alexander's Care of the Patient in Surgery. (2011, 14th ed.), Chapter 2: Concepts basic to perioperative nursing.

Perioperative Standards and Recommended Practices. (2013),
- Recommended practices for perioperative health care information management.
- Recommended practices for transfer of patient care information.
- Recommended practices for medication safety.

AORN. (2011). Position statement: Creating a practice environment of safety. Retrieved Feb. 21, 2013, from http://www.aorn.org/Clinical_Practice/Position_Statements/Position_Statements.aspx

Berry and Kohn's Operating Room Technique. (2013, 12th ed.), Chapter 2: Foundations of perioperative patient care standards; Chapter 3: Legal, regulatory, and ethical issues; Chapter 6: Administration of perioperative patient care services; Chapter 7: The patient: The reason for your existence; Chapter 21: Preoperative preparation of the patient.

Competency for Safe Patient Care During Operative and Invasive Procedures. (2009), Chapter 4: Legal, regulatory, and ethical considerations.

Key Words

Communication, documentation, HIPAA, National Patient Safety Goals, PNDS, regulatory agency, standardized communication tool, surgical safety checklist, The Joint Commission, WHO checklist

Activity — Search and Circle

According to the Health Insurance Portability and Accountability Act (HIPAA), personal health information includes:
- Name
- Address
- Birthdate
- Social security number
- Phone number, e-mail, fax
- Past, present, or future physical or mental health condition

Please circle the items on the schedule board that violate HIPAA regulations.

Time	Room	Patient	Dr.	Procedure/ Anesth
0730–0900	OR1	J. Brown SS# 100-98-0004	Smith	Laparoscopic cholecystectomy /General
0915–1145	OR1	J. Brown SS# 999-00-1234	Smith	Right carotid endarterectomy/General
1200–1330	OR1	Carl Johnson Patient is HIV +	Smith	Right inguinal hernia repair/Moderate Sedation
0730–0815	OR2	T. Adams Call his mom at 719-800-1623 when he's in PACU	Brats	Tonsillectomy/General
0730–0900	OR3	Shirley Mickle – e-mail postoperative instructions to smick@yahoo.org	Short	Abdominal hysterectomy /General
0915–1045	OR#3	Carol D. DOB 07/08/56	Short	Abdominal hysterectomy /General

Activity — Critical Thinking

A patient is scheduled for an exploratory laparotomy for a possible perforated viscus. When you arrive to interview the patient, you find the patient confused about the scheduled surgical procedure and he asks to speak to the surgeon. The permit has been signed, but the surgeon is not immediately available. What is the most appropriate course of action?

Case Study Activity

You document in Mrs. M.'s electronic medical record that an incident report (occurrence report) has been completed related to an incorrect suture count. From a legal standpoint, what are the ramifications of this documentation?

"Go To" Activity — Skill Building

Organizational policy should clearly identify appropriate communication strategies to be followed in sharing confidential patient information with designated family or friends by phone, in public waiting areas, and in any phase of the perioperative process. Review how your facility releases information on patient status to family members. Compare current practice to HIPAA privacy rules, found at http://www.hhs.gov/ocr/privacy/hipaa/understanding/summary/

Additional Reading/Resources

AORN. (2011). *Perioperative Nursing Data Set* (3rd ed.). Denver: AORN, Inc.

Centers for Medicare and Medicaid Services (CMS). (2012). The HIPAA law and related information. Retrieved Feb. 22, 2013, from http://www.cms.gov/Regulations-and-Guidance/HIPAA-Administrative-Simplification/HIPAAGenInfo/TheHIPAALawand Related-Information.html

The Joint Commission. (2013). Facts about the Universal Protocol. Retrieved Feb. 21, 2013, from http://www.jointcommission.org/standards_information/up.aspx

The Joint Commission. (2012). Facts about the official "Do Not Use" List of Abbreviations. Retrieved Feb. 21, 2013, from http://www.jointcommission.org/facts_about_the_official_/

U.S. Dept. of Health and Human Services (HHS). Health information privacy. Retrieved Feb. 21, 2013, from http://www.hhs.gov/ocr/privacy/hipaa/administrative/securityrule/index.html

Chapter Summary

Communication is an essential component of multidisciplinary practice. The effectiveness of each professional's decisions and interventions depends on the information he or she has received. Clear, consistent, and comprehensive communication with the patient, family, and all members of the multidisciplinary team facilitates patient safety and optimal outcomes.

As patient advocates, perioperative registered nurses have a duty to protect the patient from injury and to safeguard the patient's health, welfare, and safety. Effective communication, reporting, documentation, and compliance with established standards of practice and hospital policies can support advocacy and help ensure patient safety.

Glossary

Accountable — The state of being answerable to self, patient, profession, and agency for nursing care given.

Advance directive — A patient's signed and witnessed directive regarding health care, life-sustaining, and end-of-life decisions.

American Nurses Association (ANA) — Professional organization representing registered nurses. The ANA promulgates the Code of Ethics for nurses with interpretive statements that articulates the moral commitment to maintain the values and ethical obligations of all nurses. (www.ana.org)

Assessment — Assessment begins with data collection and ends with the formation of nursing diagnoses. It includes patient's history and physical exam findings, vital signs, and all aspects of presenting condition. Assessment is ongoing during the perioperative period (i.e., includes preoperative, intraoperative, postoperative).

Autonomy — In the context of health care, autonomy is the patient's self-determination or ability and power to make his or her own decisions regarding health care.

Communication — The transfer of information that requires a sender, a message, and a receiver. Transmission may be verbal, non-verbal, or written.

Continuum of care — Care of patients undergoing operative or other invasive procedures is planned and implemented along a continuum — from the time the decision to undergo surgery is made, through the intraoperative period, and for an undetermined postoperative period until the patient's health status is improved or a specified health goal is reached.

Culture of patient safety — An atmosphere of mutual trust in which all staff members can talk freely about safety issues and how to solve them without fear of blame or punishment. It is considered essential to the improvement of patient safety in any organization.

Demonstration and return demonstration — The act of teaching that involves the visible, active demonstration of an activity, then involving the learner by having him or her demonstrate the identical activity back to the teacher.

Discharge planning — The process of assessing the needs of patients for post-procedure care; developing a coordinated and multidisciplinary plan to provide the care required (including patient and family education, available services, and referral agencies and support groups); and evaluating the plan. The process begins before or on admission to the health care facility.

Documentation — The written record of nursing care including patient assessment; the actions taken as a result of that assessment; the plan of care developed and implemented; and the results of those actions. Documentation serves as the main, retrievable communication tool for the health care team.

Do-not-resuscitate (DNR) — A form of advance directives that outlines a patient's wishes for end-of life decisions. "Allow natural death" (AND) better represents the patient's decision not to have "heroic measures" implemented to prolong life, and may be used in place of DNR.

Evidence-based practice (EBP) — Practices with outcomes that have been validated by research.

Family — For the purposes of this guide, "family" includes significant others and extended family.

Hand off — The transfer of information (along with authority and responsibility) during transitions in care across the continuum for the purpose of ensuring the continuity and safety of the patient's care.

Health care team — The providers of patient care services who are required to provide direct patient care to help the patient achieve a positive outcome. Support services include, but are not limited to, pharmacy, radiology, blood bank, housekeeping, etc.

Health Insurance Portability and Accountability Act of 1996 (HIPAA) — Provides federal protection for personal health information, whether electronic, written, or oral. Disclosure of personal health information needed for patient care and other important purposes is permitted.

I PASS the BATON — A standardized method of organizing thoughts and communication using the following components: **I**nformation, **P**atient **A**ssessment, **S**ituation, **S**afety concerns, **B**ackground, **A**ction, **T**iming, **O**wnership, **N**ext.

The Joint Commission (TJC) — The independent accrediting organization that designates acceptable patient care and evaluates health care facilities' abilities to adhere to specific guidelines (e.g., documentation, processes, policies, and procedures). (www.jointcommission.org)

Knowledge — Defined as an organized body of information, usually of a factual or procedural nature, which, if applied, makes adequate performance of a job possible. Possession of knowledge does not ensure its proper application.

MAPS — A standardized method for organizing patient data: **M**edications; **A**llergies; **P**rocedure/**P**ertinent information; **S**pecial needs.

National Patient Safety Goals (NPSG) — Established by The Joint Commission to stimulate health care organizations' improvement processes addressing the most challenging patient safety issues.

"Never" events — Inexcusable outcomes in a health care setting.

Patient Self-Determination Act (PSDA) — Requires Medicare and Medicaid providers to give adult individuals, at the time of inpatient admission or enrollment, certain information about their rights under state laws governing advance directives.

Perioperative Nursing Data Set (PNDS) — Standardized nursing vocabulary that addresses the perioperative patient experience from pre-admission until discharge.

Protected health information (HIPAA PHI) — Any information about health status, provision of health care, or payment for health care that can be linked to a specific individual, including any part of a patient's medical record or payment history. (www.hhs.gov/ocr/privacy/hipaa/understanding/summary/index.html)

Read back — A method to decrease errors resulting from verbal communication, including verbal and telephone orders and critical lab values. The information is written down by the receiver, and is then "read back" to the sender to confirm accuracy of the message.

Root cause analysis (RCA) — Problem-solving methods aimed at identifying the root causes of problems or events. The practice of RCA is predicated on the belief that problems are best solved by attempting to correct or eliminate root causes, as opposed to merely addressing the immediately obvious symptoms.

SBAR — A standardized communication process that includes **S**ituation, **B**ackground, **A**ssessment, and **R**ecommendations. It is especially useful when there is a need to prioritize actions related to recommendations for care.

SHARED — A method of organizing thought and communication through **S**ituation; **H**istory; **A**ssessment; **R**equest; **E**valuate; **D**ocument.

Standardized communication plan — An organized method of receiving and transmitting information, usually involving a checklist and an easily remembered acronym.

Surgical Care Improvement Project (SCIP) — A CDC/CMS multi-year national campaign with the goal of substantially reducing surgical morbidity and mortality through collaborative efforts.

SURPASS — A standardized, comprehensive communication tool: **SUR**gical **PA**tient **S**afety **S**ystem.

Universal Protocol — A procedure created by The Joint Commission to prevent wrong

person, wrong procedure, wrong site surgery in hospitals and outpatient settings. The Universal Protocol consists of three steps:
1. A preoperative/preprocedure verification process
2. Marking the operative/procedure site
3. A time-out (final verification), which is performed immediately before starting the operation/procedure

WHO checklist — A surgical checklist containing items to be reviewed during crucial stages of the perioperative experience. The goal is to improve patient safety by adhering to proven standards of care.

References

American Nurses Association (ANA). (2004). *Nursing Scope and Standards of Practice.* Silver Spring, MD: ANA.

American Nurses Credentialing Center (ANCC). (2013). The Magnet Recognition Program®. Retrieved Feb. 7, 2013, from http://nursecredentialing.org/Magnet/ProgramOverview.aspx

AORN. (2011). *Perioperative Nursing Data Set* (3rd ed.). Denver: AORN, Inc.

AORN. (2011). Position statement: Creating a practice environment of safety. Retrieved Feb. 21, 2013, from http://www.aorn.org/Clinical_Practice/Position_Statements/Position_Statements.aspx

AORN. (2013). Recommended practices for transfer of patient care information. In *Perioperative Standards and Recommended Practices*. Denver: AORN, Inc.

Institute for Healthcare Improvement. (2011, June). SBAR technique for communication: A situational briefing model. Retrieved Feb. 7, 2013, from http://www.ihi.org/knowledge/Pages/Tools/SBARTechniqueforCommunicationASituationalBriefingModel.aspx

The Joint Commission. (2013, Jan.). *Comprehensive Accreditation and Certification Manual E-dition.* Retrieved Feb. 20, 2013, from https://e-dition.jcrinc.com/

The Joint Commission. (2012). *Improving America's Hospitals: The Joint Commission's Annual Report on Quality and Safety.* Retrieved Feb. 21, 2013, from http://www.jointcommission.org/annualreport.aspx

The Joint Commission. (2009). *The Joint Commission Guide to Improving Staff Communication.* Oakbrook Terrace, IL: Joint Commission Resources.

North American Nursing Diagnosis (NANDA) International. Retrieved Feb. 22, 2013, from http://www.nanda.org/Home.aspx

Phillips, N. (2013). *Berry and Kohn's Operating Room Technique* (12th ed.). St. Louis: Mosby.

Phippen, M. L., Ulmer, B.C., & Wells, M.P. (2009). *Competency for Safe Patient Care During Operative and Invasive Procedures.* Denver: CCI.

Rothrock, J.C. (Ed.). (2011). *Alexander's Care of the Patient in Surgery* (14th ed.). St. Louis: Mosby.

Answers to Chapter 4 Activities

Module I: Verbal and nonverbal communication — Pages 143-147

Activity — Short Answer

For each closed-ended (directive) preoperative interview question, provide an associated open-ended (non-directive) question. Compare the differences in quality and quantity of information received utilizing both approaches.

Sample responses:
1. When was the last time you had anything to eat or drink?
2. Tell me what your name is.
3. In your own words, tell me what type of surgery you're having.
4. What else can I help you with?

Source: Phillips, N. (2013). *Berry and Kohn's Operating Room Technique* (12th ed., pp. 374-378). St. Louis: Mosby.

Case Study Activity

1. What part of Mrs. M.'s assessment requires an immediate intervention?

Low potassium level.

2. Use the SBAR (Situation, Background, Assessment, Recommendation) format to describe how you would communicate this information to the surgeon and anesthesia care provider.

Sample response:
S = Your patient, Mrs. M., has a preoperative potassium level of 3.1.
B = She has a history of hypertension and currently takes hydrochlorothiazide 25 mg every day. She took her usual meds this morning with a sip of water.
A = Her EKG shows u waves and a flattened T wave indicating hypokalemia.
R = I've placed her on an EKG monitor and have notified the front desk and her family that the case may be delayed until you see her. I'd like you to come and assess Mrs. M. now. I will have potassium and an IV infusion pump available. Is there anything else you'll need?

Source: Rothrock, J.C. (Ed.). *Alexander's Care of the Patient in Surgery.* (2011, 14th ed., p. 31). St. Louis: Mosby.

Activity — Critical Thinking

1. Highlight the areas in the scenario in which breaks in communication or protocol influenced patient outcomes. Then compare those areas with the analysis of the discussion below.

- *Verifying the correct surgical site at the time of surgery is the responsibility of not only preoperative registered nurses but every member of the health care team.*

- *Active involvement and effective communication are essential to ensure continuity, safety, and quality. Using a standardized check list concurrently with a time-out is now considered best practice in preventing wrong patient, site, and side surgery.*

- *Policies and procedures should define who is responsible for marking the surgical site and how the Universal Protocol is implemented. The Joint Commission recommends that the person performing the procedure should mark the site, which did not happen in this case.*

- *Multiple checks can help identify if any discrepancies exist among the history and physical exam findings, surgical consent, patient's verbal acknowledgement, and x-ray films. Consistent implementation was not evident in this case, and an error in placing the x-rays on the viewfinder, in which the films were put up backward, went undetected.*

- *Marking of the surgical site and side should be visible after the patient has been prepped and draped. The field was prepped and draped before the surgeon arrived in the OR, and no obvious site or side markings were noted.*

- *The surgeon reviewed the appropriate patient films and abruptly requested that the nurse move the ESU and bipolar cautery pedals to the other side, which was in direct conflict with the physician's preference card and longstanding history of where the surgeon preferred the control pedals for a left-sided laminectomy. The nurse thought this was highly unusual, but did not raise her concerns with the surgeon who appeared in a hurry and distracted. The pedals were moved, no further questions were raised, and appropriate dialogue did not occur.*

- *The nurse left the room briefly to retrieve sutures, and when she returned, the anesthesiologist confirmed that the time-out had occurred during her absence. The nurse documented in the operative record that the time-out took place, although she had not directly witnessed or participated in the process. It is everyone's responsibility to participate in the time-out, and priorities should have prevented the nurse from leaving the room to retrieve suture until after the time-out. In addition, documentation of the time-out should have been completed by the anesthesiologist or surgeon who was present and who actively participated in the process. The nurse made a serious documentation error and created an ethical dilemma. By completing the time-out checklist and signing her name, she unwittingly falsified the patient's operative record.*

- *Due to the size of the incision and the failure of the surgical team to identify the actual operative side, the wrong-side surgery was not detected until the surgeon completed the procedure and was reviewing the records and documenting the postoperative orders. Only at this time did the team become aware that the surgery had been performed on the wrong side.*

2. What should be done to prevent the above situation from reoccurring?

- ***Perform a root cause analysis (RCA) to reveal the variables that contributed to this wrong-side surgery, including failed communication.***
- ***Revise the policy for wrong site, wrong procedure, and wrong person surgery.***
- ***Provide education to all members of the surgical team on the importance of active involvement and open communication by all members of the health care team.***
- ***Perform regular audits to ensure adherence to the revised policy.***

Source: Rothrock, J.C. (Ed.). *Alexander's Care of the Patient in Surgery*. (2011, 14th ed., p. 31). St. Louis: Mosby.

Activity — Critical Thinking

As she leaves the room to get additional suture, the circulating nurse asks the student she is precepting to put sterile saline in the basin opened on the ring stand. When she returns, she sees an unopened bottle of sterile saline sitting in the basin. How could this situation have been avoided?

- ***Provide clearer instructions, such as, "Pour the sterile saline into the sterile basin, standing far enough away from the basin to avoid contaminating the field. Do not allow the saline to splash out of the basin."***
- ***The circulator should not have delegated this task to the student without first evaluating her competence in transferring liquids to the sterile field.***

Source: Rothrock, J.C. (Ed.). (2011). *Alexander's Care of the Patient in Surgery* (14th ed., p.10). St. Louis: Mosby.

Module 2: Written communication — Pages 147-150

Activity — Search and Circle

Please circle the items on the schedule board that violate HIPAA regulations.

Time	Room	Patient	Dr.	Procedure/ Anesth
0730-0900	OR1	J. Brown SS# 100-98-0004	Smith	Laparoscopic cholecystectomy / General
0915-1145	OR1	J. Brown SS# 999-00-1234	Smith	Right carotid endarterectomy/General
1200-1330	OR1	Carl Johnson Patient is HIV +	Smith	Right inguinal hernia repair/Moderate Sedation
0730-0815	OR2	T. Adams Call his mom at 719-800-1623 when he's in PACU	Brats	Tonsillectomy/General
0730-0900	OR3	Shirley Mickle – e-mail postoperative instructions to smick@yahoo.org	Short	Abdominal hysterectomy /General
0915-1045	OR#3	Carol D. DOB 07/08/56	Short	Abdominal hysterectomy /General

Source: U.S. Dept of Health and Human Services (2003, May). Summary of the HIPAA Privacy Rule. Retrieved Feb. 7, 2013, from http://www.hhs.gov/ocr/privacy/hipaa/understanding/summary/

Activity — Critical Thinking

A patient is scheduled for an exploratory laparotomy for a possible perforated viscus. When you arrive to interview the patient, you find the patient confused about the scheduled surgical procedure and he asks to speak to the surgeon. The permit has been signed, but the surgeon is not immediately available. What is the most appropriate course of action?

The patient should not be transported to the OR until the surgeon has answered questions to the patient's satisfaction.

Source: Phillips, N. (2013). *Berry and Kohn's Operating Room Technique* (12th ed., pp. 45-47). St. Louis: Mosby.

Case Study Activity

You document in Mrs. M.'s electronic medical record that an incident report (occurrence report) has been completed related to an incorrect suture count. From a legal standpoint, what are the ramifications of this documentation?

The contents of a patient's medical record are discoverable in a court of law. Incident or occurrence reports are considered part of the overall institution/department quality improvement initiative and constitute privileged, private information. The fact that an incident report was filled out should not be documented in the patient's permanent record.

Source: Phillips, N. (2013). *Berry and Kohn's Operating Room Technique* (12th ed., p. 50). St. Louis: Mosby.

CHAPTER 5:
Transfer of Care

Test Specifications:
5% of CNOR test questions are based on Transfer of Care.

Introduction

Patient transfer, also called patient hand-off, involves passing care of the patient from one health care professional to another. Transfers occur many times during a patient's stay, regardless of the type of facility or setting. The goal of patient transfer is seamless continuity of care — a hallmark of patient safety. The increase in same day surgery, shorter hospital stays, and an older and higher acuity patient population increase the potential for errors related to transfer.

This chapter will help you develop a plan that actively involves staff members, patients, and their families in the transfer process. Implementing a multi-disciplinary approach to every phase of patient care is emphasized. The importance of postoperative patient education is stressed.

Module 1: Transfer of Care Between Team Members

Though it may seem a simple task to hand over responsibility for a patient from one caregiver to another, patient transfer is a complex process. Omissions in vital information may contribute to adverse outcomes. A transfer may or may not involve moving the patient from one place to another, but it always involves identifying and communicating the information required for continuity of care. The complexity of a transfer process increases when the nurse must gather information needed by colleagues in several disciplines who manage different aspects of the patient's care.

Competency Outcomes

To successfully complete the activities in this module, you will need to be able to:

1. Identify the components of transfer of patient care pre-, intra-, and postoperatively.
2. Use a standardized reporting process for communicating pertinent patient information to the next health care provider.

Recommended Reading

Alexander's Care of the Patient in Surgery. (2011, 14th ed.), Chapter 2: Patient safety and risk management; Unit II: Surgical interventions.

Perioperative Standards and Recommended Practices. (2013), Recommended practices: Transfer of patient care information.

Berry and Kohn's Operating Room Technique. (2013, 12th ed.), Chapter 11: Ambulatory surgery centers and alternative surgical locations; Chapter 25: Coordinated roles of the scrub person and the circulating nurse; Chapter 30: Postoperative patient care.

Competency for Safe Patient Care During Operative and Invasive Procedures. (2009), Chapter 6: Transfer the patient.

Key Words

Communication, continuity of care, hand-off, multidisciplinary, transfer of care

Activity — Multiple Choice

For each of the following components related to transfer of care, identify in which phase of care this information should be provided. Some answers will be used more than once.

1. Verification of correct patient, site, and procedure ____

2. Surgical count status ____

3. Allergies ____

4. Precautions (transmission based, latex allergy, etc.) ____

5. Complications associated with this surgery ____

6. Specimens ____

7. Communication with family ____

8. Required legal and clinical documentation (e.g., history & physical, informed consent) __

9. Risk for development of hypothermia ____

10. Thermal interventions ____

11. Thermal status ____

A = Preoperative

B = Intraoperative

C = Postoperative

Case Study Activity

Many facilities have developed a "hand-off" form for transferring patient information from one level of care to another. What information related to Mrs. M. should be included in your hand-off to:

A. The circulating nurse who relieves you for lunch:

B. The PACU nurse assigned to care for your patient:

Additional Readings/Resources

Amato-Vealey, E.J. (2008). Hand-off communication: A requisite for perioperative patient safety. *AORN Journal, 88*(5), 763-774.

Clancy, C.M. (2008). The importance of simulation: Preventing hand-off mistakes. *AORN Journal, 88*(4), 625-627.

The Joint Commission. (2010). *Advancing Effective Communication, Cultural Competence, and Patient- and Family-Centered Care: A Roadmap for Hospitals*. Oakbrook Terrace, IL: The Joint Commission. Retrieved Feb. 25, 2013, from http://www.jointcommission.org/assets/1/6/ARoadmap forHospitalsfinalversion727.pdf.

Micheli, A.J., Curran-Campbell, S., & Connor, L. (2010). The evolution of a surgical liaison program in a children's hospital. *AORN Journal, 92*(2), 158-168.

Stefan, K.A. (2010). The nurse liaison in perioperative services: A family-centered approach. *AORN Journal, 92*(2), 150-157.

"Go To" Activity — Skill Building

Review how your facility updates families on a family member's progress in the OR/procedural area.

Represent your perioperative department by participating in patient rounds.

Compare your facility's current practice on communicating patient care information with AORN's recommended practices for transfer of patient care information.

Module 2: Discharge Planning for the Patient Leaving the Facility

The patient and family are entitled to discharge planning services that are appropriate and individualized to their needs. Federal and state requirements may affect specific components of the discharge plan. The discharge plan must address any required follow-up services (e.g., supervision, support services, physical therapy, etc.); information about medications prescribed and how to use them appropriately; and when and how to contact a health care provider. In addition to rights, patients also have the responsibility to participate as fully as possible in the discharge planning process; the perioperative nurse should encourage this whenever it is feasible.

Competency Outcomes

To successfully complete the activities in this module, you will need to be able to:

1. Incorporate recommended standards and regulatory requirements into discharge planning.
2. Provide patient and family postoperative education based on assessed needs.

Recommended Reading

Alexander's Care of the Patient in Surgery. (2011, 14th ed.), Chapter 9: Postoperative patient care and pain management; Chapter 25: Pediatric surgery; Chapter 26: Geriatric surgery.

Berry and Kohn's Operating Room Technique. (2013, 12th ed.), Chapter 11: Ambulatory surgery centers and alternative surgical locations; Chapter 30: Perianesthesia and post-procedural patient care.

Competency for Safe Patient Care During Operative and Invasive Procedures. (2009), Chapter 18: Facilitate care after the procedure; Chapter 37: Care of the pediatric patient; Chapter 38: Care of the geriatric patient.

Key Words

Collaboration, discharge planning, education, health literacy, multidisciplinary, pain management, regulatory guidelines, wound care

Activity — Short Answer

The Joint Commission's *Comprehensive Accreditation Manual for Hospitals* (CAMH) outlines the scope of responsibilities health care organizations have for discharge planning needs for all patients, including those who have undergone operative and invasive procedures. Two core elements identified are arranging and assisting in arranging the services needed by the patient after discharge. Activities related to those core elements that are associated with discharge planning include teaching patients what they need to know about their care, treatment, and services as well as coordinating those key elements when the patient is referred, transferred, or discharged. Thus, even though the nurse-patient interaction may be brief and focused, there is a clear role for the perioperative nurse to meet the needs of the patient and family and to maintain the continuity of care, treatment, and services.

Activities related to The Joint Commission discharge planning needs include:

1. ____

2. ____

Activity — Fill in the Blanks

A patient who has undergone a procedure involving moderate sedation/analgesia should be able to stay awake for at least ____________________________ (length of time) without stimulation before being considered ready for discharge.

A patient with a malignant hyperthermia (MH) crisis should be observed in a critical care setting a minimum of ____________________________ (length of time) after the MH crisis.

Activity — Critical Thinking

1. You are employed in an office-based surgery setting. What general discharge instructions should be provided for a healthy 26-year-old woman who has just had a small lipoma removed from her left forearm?

2. How would your answer to question #1 above differ if your patient was a 5-year-old girl who had just had an umbilical herniorraphy?

Case Study Activity

Mrs. M.'s husband's primary language is Spanish. He would like to help Mrs. M. with her care after she returns home from the hospital. How can you assist him in understanding Mrs. M.'s discharge instructions?

Activity — Critical Thinking

PZ, a 55-year-old woman, is scheduled to undergo repair of a torn left rotator cuff as an ambulatory procedure. She is the sole caretaker for her frail, elderly mother who lives with her. PZ states that it is important to both of them that her mother remains at home.

PZ injured her shoulder assisting her mother with routine activities of daily living (ADLs) and delayed seeing a surgeon because of her caretaker responsibilities. As a consequence, she is quite uncomfortable and rates the level of her pain as an 8 on a scale of 0 to 10. She is looking forward to having the repair done so that she can regain lost function and reduce or eliminate her shoulder pain. However, she worries about how her recovery will affect her ability to care for her mother.

PZ is 5 feet tall and weighs 165 pounds. She smokes one pack of cigarettes per day and was diagnosed a year ago with obstructive sleep apnea (OSA). PZ reports that she has difficulty wearing the continuous positive airway pressure (CPAP) mask that she was given when her OSA was diagnosed. She also has elevated blood pressure, but it is managed with medication. She reports that she can become sleepy during the day and often must take naps.

1. When should discharge planning begin?

2. How does PZ's diagnosis of OSA influence the planned procedure?

3. What immediate goals should be addressed in the discharge plan of care, and how can they be approached in a multidisciplinary manner with PZ?

4. What are the educational needs associated with PZ's postoperative plan of care, and how should this information be presented?

"Go To" Activity — Skill Building

Volunteer to talk with patients and their families about their surgical experiences during hospital tours or preoperative visits.

Assist with follow-up phone calls to discharged patients. What are the most frequent questions, concerns, and complications voiced by your patients? How can this information be incorporated to improve care for future patients?

Talk with a case manager or social worker about his or her job. Incorporate discharge planning into the perioperative plan of care by anticipating and addressing potential problems with the appropriate discipline.

Additional Reading/Resources

Flanagan, J. (2009). Postoperative telephone calls: Timing is everything. *AORN Journal, 90*(1), 41-51.

The Joint Commission. (2012, June). *Hot topics in health care, Transitions of care: The need for a more effective approach to continuing patient care.* Retrieved Feb. 25, 2013, from http://www.jointcommission.org/assets/1/18/Hot_Topics_Transitions_of_Care.pdf

Monachos, C.L. (2007). Assessing and addressing low health literacy among surgical outpatients. *AORN Journal, 90*(2), 373-383.

Taylor, E. (2009). Providing developmentally based care for preschoolers. *AORN Journal, 88*(2), 267-273.

Taylor, E. (2009). Providing developmentally based care for school-aged and adolescent patients. *AORN Journal, 90*(2), 261-267.

Taylor, E. (2008). Providing developmentally based care for toddlers. *AORN Journal, 87*(5), 992-999.

Chapter Summary

Effective discharge planning for the patient undergoing an operative or invasive procedure is an evolving process, starting when the patient agrees to undergo the procedure and ending when recovery is complete. A well-planned, thorough, standardized transfer process based on patient needs is more consistently implemented regardless of setting.

The perioperative nurse contributes to the discharge plan of care by identifying appropriate desired outcomes related to the patient and the procedure, and by collaborating with other members of the health care team to help the patient and family achieve those outcomes as fully as possible. Appropriate and effective discharge planning is a key component of returning the patient to an optimal level of wellness.

Glossary

Ambulatory surgery — For purposes of this guide, "ambulatory surgery" includes outpatient surgery, same-day surgery, day surgery, etc.

Discharge planning — The process of assessing the needs of patients for post-procedure care, developing a coordinated and multidisciplinary plan to provide the care required (including patient and family education, available services, and referral agencies and support groups), and evaluating the plan. The process begins before or on admission to the health care facility.

Documentation — The written record of nursing care including patient assessment, the actions taken as a result of that assessment, the plan of care developed and implemented, and the results of those actions. Documentation serves as the main, retrievable communication tool for the health care team.

Family — For purposes of this guide, "family" includes significant others and extended family.

Health literacy — The ability to apply information in making health care decisions.

Interdisciplinary collaboration — A process of joint decision making and communication among health care providers with the mutual goal of satisfying the needs of the patient while respecting the unique abilities of each person involved in the care. Trust, knowledge, mutual respect, cooperation, coordination, shared responsibility, good communication skills, and optimism are desired traits of the multidisciplinary team.

National Patient Safety Goals — Established in 2002 by The Joint Commission to help accredited organizations address specific areas of concern in regards to patient safety.

Outcome criteria — Statements developed to identify the tasks or conditions to be implemented that will assist the patient in achieving the desired outcomes. Outcome criteria indicate an expected, measurable change in the patient's health status.

*Perioperative Nursing Data Set: The Perioperative Nursing Vocabulary (*PNDS) — A guidebook that provides nursing diagnoses, nursing interventions, and patient outcomes statements specific to the perioperative environment.

References

AORN. (2011). *Perioperative Nursing Data Set* (3rd ed.). Denver: AORN, Inc.

AORN. (2013). *Perioperative Standards and Recommended Practices*. Denver: AORN, Inc.

The Joint Commission. (2013). *Comprehensive Accreditation Manual for Hospitals: The Official Handbook,* PC 04.01.01. Oakbrook Terrace, IL: The Joint Commission.

Phillips, N. (2013). *Berry and Kohn's Operating Room Technique*. (12th ed.). St. Louis: Mosby.

Phippen, M.L., Ulmer, B.C., & Wells, M.P. (2009). *Competency for Safe Patient Care During Operative and Invasive Procedures*. Denver: CCI.

Rothrock, J.C. (Ed.). (2011). *Alexander's Care of the Patient in Surgery* (14th ed.). St. Louis: Mosby.

Answers to Chapter 5 Activities

Module 1: Transfer of care between team members — Pages 159-161

Activity — Multiple Choice

For each of the following components related to transfer of care, identify in which phase of care this information should be provided. Some answers will be used more than once.

      A = preoperative   *B = intraoperative*   *C = postoperative*

1. Verification of correct patient, site, and procedure: *A, B, C*

2. Surgical count status: *B*

3. Allergies: *A, B, C*

4. Precautions (transmission based, latex allergy, etc.): *A, B, C*

5. Complications associated with this surgery: *C*

6. Specimens: *B*

7. Communication with family: *A, B, C*

8. Required legal and clinical documentation (e.g., history and physical, informed consent): *A*

9. Risk for development of hypothermia: *A*

10. Thermal interventions: *B*

11. Thermal status: *C*

> Source: AORN. (2013). Recommended practices for transfer of patient care information, pp. 446-447. In *Perioperative Standards and Recommended Practices*. Denver: AORN, Inc.

Case Study Activity

Many facilities have developed a "hand-off" form for transferring patient information from one level of care to another. What information related to Mrs. M. should be included in your hand-off to:

A. The circulating nurse who relieves you for lunch:

Sample responses:
Name of patient, procedure, history of diabetes, hypertension, allergy to PCN, suspected latex allergy, suspected MH, current count, current meds on field, location of any additional supplies, current status of counts, update on any additional personnel needed (radiology technician,

moving assistance, etc.), specimens, last blood glucose reading.

B. The PACU nurse assigned to care for your patient:

Name of patient, name of surgeon, procedure, name of anesthesia care provider, type of anesthetic, history of diabetes, hypertension, description of home medications, allergy to PCN, suspected latex allergy, suspected MH, total IV fluids, estimated blood loss, location of IV site/patency, any meds given including pain meds, vital signs, blood glucose values including time of last finger stick, site and condition of dressings/drains, sequential compression stockings, thermal interventions in OR.

Source: Rothrock, J.C. (Ed.). (2011). *Alexander's Care of the Patient in Surgery* (14th ed., p. 31). St. Louis: Mosby.

Module 2: Discharge planning for the patient leaving the facility — Pages 162-166

Activity — Short Answer

Activities related to The Joint Commission's discharge planning needs include:

1. Teaching patients what they need to know about care, treatment, and services.
2. Coordinating services when patient is referred, transferred, or discharged.

Source: The Joint Commission. (2013). *Comprehensive Accreditation Manual for Hospitals: The Official Handbook*, PC 04.01.05, PC 65, 66. Oakbrook Terrace, IL: The Joint Commission.

Activity — Fill in the Blanks

A patient who has undergone a procedure involving moderate sedation/analgesia should be able to stay awake for at least ***20 minutes*** without stimulation before being considered ready for discharge.

Source: AORN. (2013). Recommended practices for managing the patient receiving moderate sedation/analgesia, p. 419. In *Perioperative Standards and Recommended Practices*. Denver: AORN, Inc.

A patient with a malignant hyperthermia crisis should be observed in a critical care setting a minimum of ***36 hours*** after the MH crisis.

Source: Malignant Hyperthermia Association of the United States (MHAUS). (2011). *Anesthetics*. Retrieved Feb. 5, 2013, from http://www.mhaus.org/anesthetics/

Activity — Critical Thinking

1. You are employed in an office-based surgery setting. What general discharge instructions should be provided for a healthy 26-year-old woman who has just had a small lipoma removed from her left forearm?

Pain control methods, both pharmacologic and non-pharmacologic; wound and dressing care; activity level; side effects of any medications ordered; signs and symptoms of infection; when and who to contact for additional assistance/questions/concerns; when to return to the office for suture removal; any other information based on specific patient needs.

Source: Rothrock, J.C. (Ed.). (2011). *Alexander's Care of the Patient in Surgery.* (14th ed., p. 292). St. Louis: Mosby.

2. How would your answer to question #1 above differ if your patient was a 5-year-old girl who had just had an umbilical herniorraphy?

The parents or guardians will be included in postoperative teaching. Activity restrictions include when the child could return to school or day care and any limitations on running or physical contact while playing. Demonstrate wound care on a stuffed animal or doll. Allow the child to handle any objects that will be used in care (e.g., temporal or tympanic membrane thermometer). Identify the method the child will use to communicate pain (words like "ouch" or "owie") and/or the use of a pain scale such as FACES. Put a similar dressing or band-aid on the child's personal stuffed animal or toy. Encourage fluids and easy-to-digest foods. The child may exhibit increased separation anxiety or regression immediately after the procedure and require additional comfort measures from caregivers. Use popular cartoon, movie, or storybook characters and terminology to help describe experiences and reinforce postoperative teaching.

Sources: Rothrock, J.C. (Ed.). (2011). *Alexander's Care of the Patient in Surgery.* (14th ed., pp.1086-1098). St. Louis: Mosby; Phillips, N. (2013). *Berry and Kohn's Operating Room Technique,* pp. 127-135, 159. St. Louis: Mosby; Phippen, M.L., Ulmer, B.C., & Wells, M.P. (2009). *Competency for Safe Patient Care During Operative and Invasive Procedures*, pp. 1311-1318. Denver: CCI.

Case Study Activity

Mrs. M.'s husband's primary language is Spanish. He would like to help Mrs. M. with her care after she returns home from the hospital. How can you assist him in understanding Mrs. M.'s discharge instructions?

Information should be provided to Mr. M. in an understandable form. This may include written literature in Spanish, models, diagrams, or drawings. Consider using an interpreter or an electronic method of interpretation/translation. The nurse must remember that teaching is only complete when the patient and family are able to either teach back or verbalize understanding of what has been covered.

Source: Rothrock, J.C. (Ed.). (2011). *Alexander's Care of the Patient in Surgery.* (14th ed., p. 292). St. Louis: Mosby.

Activity — Critical Thinking

PZ, a 55-year-old woman, is scheduled to undergo repair of a torn left rotator cuff as an ambulatory procedure. She is the sole caretaker for her frail, elderly mother who lives with her. PZ states that it is important to both of them that her mother remains at home.

PZ injured her shoulder assisting her mother with routine activities of daily living (ADLs) and delayed seeing a surgeon because of her caretaker responsibilities. As a consequence, she is quite uncomfortable and rates the level of her pain as an 8 on a scale of 0 to 10. She is looking forward to having the repair done so that she can regain lost function and reduce or eliminate her shoulder pain. However, she worries about how her recovery will affect her ability to care for her mother.

PZ is 5 feet tall and weighs 165 pounds. She smokes one pack of cigarettes per day and was diagnosed a year ago with obstructive sleep apnea (OSA). PZ reports that she has difficulty wearing the continuous positive airway pressure (CPAP) mask that she was given when her OSA was diagnosed. She also has elevated blood pressure, but it is managed with medication. She reports that she can become sleepy during the day and often must take naps.

1. When should discharge planning begin?

Discharge planning for PZ should begin in the surgeon's office when she agrees to have her rotator cuff repaired.

2. How does PZ's diagnosis of OSA influence the planned procedure?

PZ's OSA diagnosis is significant because it may affect her ability to have the procedure done on an ambulatory basis, and it will influence the type of anesthesia selected. She should plan on being monitored in the hospital overnight to prevent poor outcomes. The surgeon's office staff may need to work with PZ's insurer to obtain precertification for admission to avoid possible cancellation of her procedure.

3. What immediate goals should be addressed in the discharge plan of care, and how can they be approached in a multidisciplinary manner with PZ?

PZ's immediate goals for discharge planning would include:
1. Pain management and control to an acceptable level
2. Prevention of postoperative infection
3. Return to optimal function
4. Address mother's needs in terms of home care or short-term stay in assisted living facility
5. Maintenance of current home meds to control hypertension

Secondary goals include weight loss and smoking cessation counseling; respite care as needed for mother; re-evaluation of CPAP mask fit.

These goals are addressed by a variety of caregivers, including physicians, nutritionists, social workers, and nurses.

4. What are the educational needs associated with PZ's postoperative plan of care, and how should this information be presented?

The educational needs associated with PZ's situation are primarily focused on pain management, wound healing, and regaining function. Pharmacologic and nonpharmacologic approaches to managing pain and realistic expectations for long-term pain control should be reviewed in terms that PZ can easily understand. Providing information in a variety of formats

(verbal, written, video, etc.) will aid in retention of material. Signs and symptoms of wound infection should be reviewed, along with information on how smoking negatively affects wound healing and increases the risk for infection. Part of the recovery process for PZ will be regaining function in her shoulder, so she must clearly understand any prescribed postoperative exercises and set up an appointment for physical therapy after the procedure.

CHAPTER 6:
Cleaning, Disinfecting, Packaging, Sterilizing, Transporting, and Storing Instruments and Supplies

Test Specifications:
12% of CNOR test questions are based on Cleaning, Disinfecting, Packaging, Sterilizing, Transporting, and Storing Instruments and Supplies.

Introduction

The defining characteristic of the perioperative arena is its sterile environment that protects patients during surgical procedures. The perioperative nurse has the unique responsibility to create a sterile field and ensure its continued sterility until the patient's skin integrity is restored and he/she is safe from harm from exposure to pathogens. Appropriate sterilization and disinfection of instruments and equipment in that sterile field protect both patients and perioperative personnel from exposure to infectious material.

Disinfection and sterilization is an area where the professional perioperative nurse understands the interactive nature of a multidisciplinary environment and how one discipline can influence the effectiveness of another. Although the disinfection and sterilization of instruments is usually done in a sterile processing department (SPD), perioperative nurses participate actively in ensuring that the instruments and equipment are effectively processed. Processing of instruments and equipment begins at the point of use. Everyone who handles sterile instrumentation and equipment participates in the process.

The perioperative nurse who has knowledge of the principles and practices involved in infection prevention, and the legal and regulatory requirements that impact the practice, is well prepared to think critically and make effective practice decisions about cleaning, disinfecting, packaging, sterilizing, transporting, and storing instruments and supplies.

This chapter will challenge your critical thinking and decision-making skills related to current infection prevention and disinfection and sterilization practices. Applying these principles and practices will help you protect your patient and reduce the risk of surgical site infections. This chapter will also prepare you to ensure the sterility of instruments and equipment delivered to the sterile field regardless of where they were processed.

Module 1: Microbiological Considerations Related to Infection Control Principles

Introduction

Any microorganism can be pathogenic if it invades a susceptible area. The skin and mucous membranes are the body's primary protection against infection.

The most common source of pathogens found in surgical site infections is the patient's own flora (CDC, 1999); however, pathogens can be introduced onto the sterile field from other sources, including contaminated instruments, supplies, or other people. Proper sterilization and disinfection practices disrupt the chain of infection by removing pathogens.

Perioperative personnel also are at risk for exposure to pathogens. Personal protective equipment and good aseptic technique protect personnel from contamination and infection. Studies have demonstrated that double-gloving can reduce personnel exposure to pathogens via needlesticks (AORN, 2013, pp.97-98).

In addition to the common infectious agents encountered in the OR, there are always new and challenging microorganisms. Microorganisms that have developed resistance to common antibiotics have evolved into pathogens such as methicillin-resistant *Staphylococcus aureus* (MRSA), vancomycin-resistant *Enterococcus* (VRE), and multidrug-resistant *Mycobacterium tuberculosis* (MDR-TB) that require special attention. The prion that causes Creutzfeld-Jacob disease (CJD) is not destroyed using routine procedures for disinfection and sterilization of surgical instruments. We will continue to be challenged to protect our patients and ourselves as microorganisms adapt to our efforts to eradicate them.

Competency Outcomes

To successfully complete the activities in this module, you will need to be able to:

1. Choose appropriate personal protective equipment (PPE) required to reduce the risk of transmitting infectious organisms.
2. Describe the proper management of patients with known or suspected transmissible infections.

Recommended Readings

Alexander's Care of the Patient in Surgery. (2011, 14th ed.), Chapter 3: Infection prevention and control in the perioperative setting.

Perioperative Standards and Recommended Practices. (2013), Recommended practices:
- High level disinfection.

- Prevention of transmissible infections.

Berry and Kohn's Operating Room Technique. (2013, 12th ed.), Chapter 14: Surgical microbiology and antimicrobial therapy; Chapter 15: Principles of asepsis and sterile technique; Chapter 16: Appropriate attire, surgical hand hygiene, and gowning and gloving.

Competency for Safe Patient Care During Operative and Invasive Procedures. (2009), Chapter 11: Provide instruments, equipment, and supplies.

Key Words

Airborne precautions, chain of infection, contact precautions, Creutzfeld-Jacob disease (CJD), droplet precautions, methicillin-resistant *Staphylococcus aureus* (MRSA), multi-drug-resistant *Mycobacterium tuberculosis* (MDR-TB), pathogen, personal protective equipment (PPE), standard precautions, transmission-based precautions, vancomycin-resistant *Enterococcus* (VRE)

Activity — Fill in the Blank

The most important component of standard precautions is _______________________.

Activity — Short Answer

What nursing interventions should be implemented while caring for a patient with each of the following transmission-based precautions?

Contact:

Airborne:

Droplet:

Activity — Stop the Spread!

For each disease, choose the appropriate transmission-based precautions and associated PPE.

Disease	Transmission-based precaution	PPE
Human immunodeficiency virus (HIV)		
Mycobacterium tuberculosis		
Hepatitis B		
Staphylococcus aureus		
Clostridium difficile		
Pseudomonas		
Varicella		
Influenza		

Activity — True or False

Using an alcohol-based hand rub is the appropriate hand sanitizing method after caring for a patient with *Clostridium difficile*.

TRUE   FALSE

Activity — Critical Thinking

You have just cared for a patient who is suspected of having Creutzfeld-Jacob disease (CJD). What is the preferred method for inactivating prions on semi-critical and critical devices?

"Go To" Activity — Check It Out!

Go to Question #16, Infection control; Question #23, Transmission-based precautions; Question #37, CJD; and Questions #48 and #49, Percutaneous injuries, Parts I and II, under the Perioperative question of the week tab on your CD for additional critical-thinking questions.

Case Study Activity

In evaluating Mrs. M., what risk factors for a surgical site infection do you find?

"Go To" Activity — Skill Building

Talk with the infection control nurse or the director of infection prevention in your facility about tracking and surveillance methods for infectious diseases and surgical site infections.

Volunteer to represent your department at your facility's infection prevention committee.

Review your department's policies and procedures on standard and transmission-based precautions. Compare them to CDC and AORN standards.

Additional Reading/Resources

Centers for Disease Control and Prevention. (1999). Guideline for prevention of surgical site infection, 20(4). Retrieved Feb. 25, 2013, from http://www.cdc.gov/hicpac/pdf/guidelines/SSI_1999.pdf

Durai, R., Ng, P.C.H., & Hoque, H. (2010). Methicillin-Resistant *Staphylococcus aureus*: An update. *AORN Journal, 91*(5), 599-609.

Freeman, S.S., Lara, G.L., Courts, M.R., Wanzer, L.J., et al. (2009). An evidence-based process for evaluating infection control policies. *AORN Journal, 89*(3), 489-507.

Lassiter, S. (2011). Preventing infection: Collaboration between surgical team members and infection preventionists. *AORN Journal, 93*(2), 287-290.

Lipke, V.L., & Hyott, A.S. (2010). Reducing surgical site infections by bundling multiple risk reduction strategies and active surveillance. *AORN Journal, 92*(3), 288-296.

Tarrac, S.E. (2008). Application of the updated CDC Isolation Guidelines for Health Care Facilities. *AORN Journal, 87*(3), 534-546.

Vasaly, F.W., & Reines, H.D. (2009). A quality committee's evaluation of surgical intervention for *Clostridium difficile* infection. *AORN Journal, 90*(2), 192-204.

Module 2: Cleaning and Disinfecting Instruments and Supplies

Introduction

The process of disinfection or sterilization starts with cleaning. An item can be clean without being sterile, but no item can be sterile without being clean. Similarly, you can clean without disinfecting, but cannot disinfect without cleaning. The risk for transmitting infection is taken into account when determining the level and type of disinfection.

Facilities often manage borrowed or consigned ("loaner") instruments. Vendors may provide instrumentation for a new procedure on a trial basis, or special instrumentation for a unique procedure. A comprehensive policy to manage loaner instruments ensures that they are received in sufficient time and are properly processed on site in the same manner as facility-owned instruments.

Competency Outcomes

To successfully complete the activities in this module, you will need to be able to:

1. Recognize the influence of professional and regulatory agencies in developing practice standards related to safe processing of surgical instruments and supplies.
2. Identify infection control principles related to the cleaning and disinfection of surgical instruments and supplies.

Recommended Readings

Alexander's Care of the Patient in Surgery. (2011, 14th ed.), Chapter 3: Infection prevention and control in the perioperative setting.

Perioperative Standards and Recommended Practices. (2013), Recommended practices:
* Cleaning and processing flexible endoscopes.
* Cleaning and care of instruments and powered equipment.
* High level disinfection.
* Sterilization.

Perioperative Standards and Recommended Practices. (2013), Guidance statement:
* Environmental responsibility.

Berry and Kohn's Operating Room Technique. (2013, 12th ed.), Chapter 17: Decontamination and disinfection.

Competency for Safe Patient Care During Operative and Invasive Procedures. (2009),

Chapter 11: Provide instruments, equipment, and supplies; Chapter 14: Monitor and control the environment.

Key Words

AAMI, bioburden, cleaning, critical item, decontamination, disinfection, documentation, enzymatic cleaner, FDA, germicide, high-level disinfection, loaner instrumentation, low-level disinfection, non-critical item, PPE, semi-critical item

Activity — Multiple Choice

The most reliable source for information regarding processing of instruments and equipment is:

A. OSHA regulations

B. TJC requirements

C. FDA protocols

D. Manufacturers' instructions

Activity — Matching

Match the item to its definition.

1. Non-critical _____
2. Semi-critical _____
3. Critical _____

A. Enters sterile tissues including the vascular system

B. Contacts non-intact skin and mucous membranes

C. Contacts intact skin or does not come in contact with the patient

Activity — Put It In Its Place

Match the following items to the potential for transmitting infection and their appropriate method of processing.

Blood pressure cuff	Laparoscope	Tourniquet cuff
Laryngoscope	Doppler	Colonoscope
Balfour retractor	Mayo stand	

Disease transmission risk	*Item(s)*	*Method of processing*
Non-critical	_____________	Low-level disinfection
Non-critical	_____________	Intermediate-level disinfection
Semi-critical	_____________	High-level disinfection
Critical	_____________	Sterilization

Activity — Do You Know?

Circle all of the following that represent proper management of instruments used during a surgical procedure.

A. Wipe instruments clean of blood and debris during the procedure with a sponge moistened with sterile saline.

B. Flush lumens to prevent bioburden from drying.

C. Isolate and mark instruments in need of repair.

D. Separate contaminated from uncontaminated items on the sterile field for return to sterile processing.

E. Soak used items in enzymatic detergent or spray to prevent drying of bioburden.

Activity — Scramble

Number the following steps in high-level disinfection in the correct order:

____Flush lumens with the disinfectant.

____Clean the instrument.

____Time the immersion cycle.

____Wear appropriate PPE.

____Document results of processing.

____Check solution for minimum effective concentration.

____Deliver to point of use without contaminating.

____Rinse with sterile water.

____Immerse instrument in disinfectant according to manufacturer's recommendations.

Activity — Short Answer

How long can an item that has been high-level disinfected be stored before use?

Activity — Critical Thinking

A surgical instrumentation vendor arrives at 0715 for your scheduled 0730 anterior/posterior spinal fusion case with a set of implants that he states "are in the process of being FDA approved and the surgeon wants to trial." The implants have been sterilized at another facility and are covered with a heavy plastic dust cover. What is your response?

"Go To" Activity — Skill Building

Locate and review the Association for the Advancement of Medical Instrumentation (AAMI), *Comprehensive Guide to Steam Sterilization and Sterility Assurance in Health Care Facilities,* in your sterile processing, infection prevention, or biomed department.

Spend an afternoon in your sterile processing department. Compare cleaning, disinfection, packaging, and sterilization methods to those outlined in AORN's standards and recommended practices.

Review your policy on loaner instrumentation and compare it with AORN's standards and recommended practices. How is compliance with this policy tracked?

Review your immediate-use sterilization log for trends; recommend purchasing additional inventory for instruments that are routinely sterilized for immediate use.

"Go To" Activity — Check It Out!

Go to Question #21, Reprocessing opened and unused supplies; Question #33, Count sheets in trays; and Question #46, TASS, under the Perioperative question of the week tab on your CD for critical-thinking exercises.

Additional Readings/Resources

Allen, G. (Ed.). (2010). Infection prevention in the perioperative setting: Zero tolerance for infections. *Perioperative Nursing Clinics, 5*(4).

Burlingame, B. (2009). Reprocessing flexible endoscopes before use. *AORN Journal, 89*(2), 403-405.

Cuming, R.G., Rocco, T.S., & McEachem, A.G. (2008). Improving compliance with Occupational Safety and Health Administration Standards. *AORN Journal, 87*(2), 347-360.

Goodman, T. (Ed.). (2010). Sterilization and disinfection for the perioperative nurse. *Perioperative Nursing Clinics, 5*(3).

Module 3: Packaging and Sterilization of Instruments and Supplies

Introduction

The choice of packaging for instruments and supplies to be delivered to the sterile field is contingent on the item to be sterilized and the method of sterilization. Steam sterilization is the oldest, safest, most economical, and best understood method of sterilization; however, low temperature sterilization is becoming more popular for items that are moisture or heat sensitive.

Immediate use (previously called "flash") sterilization refers to steam sterilizing unwrapped items using an abbreviated (no drying time) cycle for immediate use on the sterile field. The practice was intended to address accidental contamination of an instrument for which no replacement was available, but the practice expanded to include flashing entire sets between cases as an alternative to increasing inventory or to decrease turnaround time waiting for the set to be reprocessed in the SPD. The Joint Commission and regulatory agencies have developed strict guidelines for immediate use sterilization. These guidelines are reflected in AORN's *Perioperative Standards and Recommended Practices*.

Competency Outcomes

To successfully complete the activities in this module, you will need to be able to:

1. Choose the correct method of sterilization for surgical instrumentation.
2. Describe processes for packaging an item for sterilization.

Recommended Readings

Alexander's Care of the Patient in Surgery. (2011, 14th ed.), Chapter 3: Infection prevention and control in the perioperative setting; Chapter 7: Surgical modalities.

Perioperative Standards and Recommended Practices. (2013),
* Guidance statement: Role of the health care industry representative.
* Recommended practices for cleaning and care of instruments and powered equipment.
* Recommended practices for selection and use of packaging systems for sterilization.
* Recommended practices for sterilization.

Berry and Kohn's Operating Room Technique. (2013, 12th ed), Chapter 18: Sterilization.

Competency for Safe Patient Care During Operative and Invasive Procedures. (2009), Chapter 9: Establish and maintain the sterile field; Chapter 14: Monitor and control the environment.

Key Words

Dynamic air removal, gravity displacement, hydrogen peroxide gas plasma sterilization, immediate use sterilization, implants, load, prevacuum, steam, sterilization

Activity — Fill in the Blank

Complete the chart below for typical cycle times for *dynamic air removal (prevacuum)* steam sterilization.

Item	Exposure time at 270° F (132° C)	Minimum dry time	Exposure time at 275° F (135° C)	Minimum dry time
Wrapped instruments	_________	_________	_________	_________
Textile packs	_________	_________	_________	_________

Complete the chart below for typical cycle times for *gravity displacement* steam sterilization.

Item	Exposure time at 250° F (121° C)	Minimum dry time	Exposure time at 270° F (132° C)	Minimum dry time	Exposure time at 275° F (135° C)	Minimum dry time
Wrapped instruments	_______	_________	_________	_________	_________	_________
Textile packs	_______	_________	_________	_________	_________	_________

Activity — Critical Thinking

Use the autoclave tape on the right to answer the following questions.

1. What method of sterilization is this?

2. What type(s) of instruments can be processed using this method of sterilization?

3. What type(s) of monitoring should be used for this method of sterilization?

4. Under what set of circumstances should this method of sterilization be used?

5. When is it inappropriate to use this method of sterilization?

6. How should this cycle be documented?

Activity — Short Answer

What is unique about packaging for hydrogen peroxide gas plasma sterilizers?

```
=======================
=======P R E V A C=======
=======================
CYCLE   START   AT   10:53:06A
                 ON      4/06/11

CYCLE  COUNT        28827
OPERATOR ______________
  STERLIZER           VAC  S2

        STER TEMP  =   270.0F
     CONTROL TEMP  =   273.0F
        STER TIME  =   4 MIN
         DRY TIME  =   0 MIN

                          V=inHg
 - TIME            T=F    P=psig

C   10:53:06A     146.4      0P
C   10:54:05A     249.1     21P
C   10:55:19A     181.8     22V
C   10:55:39A     249.7     26P
C   10:56:59A     110.5     22V
C   10:57:15A     237.5     26P
C   10:58:31A     168.2     22V
C   10:58:46A     247.3     26P
C   11:00:02A     179.6     23V
S   11:00:40A     270.1     32P
S   11:02:40A     273.5     32P
E   11:04:40A     273.2     31P
E   11:04:55A     233.7      3P
E   11:04:56A     232.6      2P
Z   11:05:08A     207.3      0P

LOAD                    040602

     TEMP MAX  =  273.8F
     TEMP MIN  =  270.1F

CONDITION      = 7:34
STERILIZE      = 4:00
EXHAUST        = 0:29
TOTAL CYCLE    = 12:03

=======================
=      READY TO UNLOAD      =
=======================

* NOT READY            3:22:48P
DOOR UNLOCKED
```

Activity — Fill in the Blank

1. The microorganism used in biologic indicators is _________________________.

2. A limitation for using low-temperature hydrogen peroxide gas plasma sterilization is

____.

3. During sterilization of double paper-plastic pouch packages, the packages should be

placed ____.
(paper-to-paper or plastic-to-plastic).

4. Which of the following sterilization methods is NOT considered low-temperature?
   ___Steam autoclave
   ___Hydrogen peroxide gas plasma
   ___Peracetic acid
   ___Ozone

Additional Readings/Resources

AAMI. (2012). *Comprehensive guide to steam sterilization and sterility assurance in healthcare facilities.* (ANSI/AAMI ST79: 2010, A3: 2012). Arlington, Va.: AAMI.

AAMI. *Immediate-use steam sterilization.* Retrieved Feb. 27, 2013, from http://www. aami.org/publications/standards/ST79_Immediate_Use_Statement.pdf.

Carlo, A. (2008). The new era of flash sterilization. *AORN Journal, 88*(6), S68-S80.

Centers for Disease Control and Prevention. (2008). *Guideline for Disinfection and Sterilization in Healthcare Facilities.* Retrieved Feb. 7, 2013, from http://www.cdc.gov/hicpac/pdf/guidelines/Disinfection_Nov_2008.pdf. (Note: It's free!)

Huber, L. (2010). Central sterile supply department professionals: A key piece in the OR quality puzzle. *AORN Journal, 91*(3), 319-320.

Hughes, C. (2008). Sterilization: Would your facility pass a standards audit? *AORN Journal, 87*(1), 176-186.

Huter-Kunish, G.G. (2009). Processing loaner instruments in an ambulatory surgery center. *AORN Journal, 89*(5), 861-870.

IAHCSMM. Position paper on the management of loaner instrumentation. Retrieved Feb.

27, 2013, from http://www.ashcsp.org/pdfs/IAHCSMM_Position_Paper_%20Management_of_Loaner_Instrumentation_070111.pdf. (Note: It's free!)

Lucas, A. D., Chobin, N., Conner, R., Gordon E. A., et al. (2009). Steam sterilization and internal count sheets: Assessing the potential for cytotoxicity. *AORN Journal, 89*(3), 521-531.

Moore, T.K. (2009). Today's sterilizer is not your father's water heater. *AORN Journal, 90*(1), 81-92.

Morris, M. L. (2011). Sterilization in the perioperative setting. *AORN Journal, 93*(3), 411-412.

Seavey, R. (2010). Collaboration between perioperative nurses and sterile processing personnel. *AORN Journal, 91*(4), 454-462.

Spry, C. (2008). Understanding current steam sterilization recommendations and guidelines. *AORN Journal, 88*(4), 537-554.

Module 4: Principles of Transporting and Storing Sterile Supplies

Introduction

Instrumentation may be appropriately cleaned, decontaminated, disinfected, packaged, and sterilized, and still arrive at the sterile field contaminated. Transporting and storing instruments safely from the point of processing to the point of use requires the same attention to detail as any other step in the process.

Competency Outcomes

To successfully complete the activities in this module, you will need to be able to:

1. Identify safe storage principles for surgical instrumentation.
2. Select correct methods for transporting sterile supplies.

Recommended Readings

Alexander's Care of the Patient in Surgery. (2011, 14th ed.), Chapter 3: Infection prevention and control in the perioperative setting.

Perioperative Standards and Recommended Practices. (2013), Recommended practices:
- Cleaning and care of instruments and powered equipment.
- Cleaning and processing endoscopes.
- Selection and use of packaging systems for sterilization.
- Sterilization.

Berry and Kohn's Operating Room Technique. (2013, 12th ed.), Chapter 18: Sterilization.

Competency for Safe Patient Care During Operative and Invasive Procedures. (2009), Chapter 9: Establish and maintain the sterile field; Chapter 14: Monitor and control the environment.

Key Words

Controlled conditions, event related, shelf life, storage, time related, transportation

Activity — Know Your Numbers

Sterile items should be stored at least _________ inches above the floor, at least __________

inches below sprinkler heads, and at least ___________ inches from outside walls.

Activity — Fill in the Blank

Shelf life of a packaged sterile item is ___________________ (time related or event related).

Activity — Multiple Choice

A flexible endoscope should be high-level disinfected before use if it has been unused for

      A. one day.
      B. three days.
      C. five days.
      D. it is not necessary for endoscopes to be high-level disinfected.

Activity — Critical Thinking

You send an orderly to pick up a pacemaker battery that has just been delivered to the receiving area of central services. The battery is in a sealed, sterile package and is still in its cardboard shipping carton. You are busy, so the orderly places the carton on a prep table inside the room.

What action should be taken?

Case Study Activity

Your scrub person has requested that you open the basic major pan for Mrs. M.'s case in anticipation of an open cholecystectomy. You bring in the wrapped pan of instruments and open it appropriately on a small table. As you remove the lid, you notice beads of water on the inside of the tray. The chemical indicator is present, and its color change indicates effective steam penetration. The tray was in its customary location in the sterile supply room.

1. Are the instruments sterile?

2. What are your options?

3. What is the significance of the load cycle lot number in this instance?

Additional Readings/Resources

Blanchard, J. (2009). Humidity, temperature, and air exchanges in the OR. *AORN Journal, 89*(6), 1129-1131.

Denholm, B. (2009). CMS requirements for sterile storage expiration dates in ASCs. *AORN Journal, 89*(5), 914-916.

Module 5: Principles of Biological and Chemical Monitoring

Introduction

Multiple methods are available for ensuring that instruments have been exposed to an environment conducive to destroying microorganisms. Biological and chemical integrators provide other quality assurance indicators that sterile instruments are being delivered to the surgical field.

Competency Outcomes

To successfully complete the activities in this module, you will need to be able to:

1. Differentiate between physical, chemical, and biologic indicators.
2. Identify appropriate uses for Class 1, 2, 3, 4, and 5 indicators.
3. Evaluate sterilization monitoring practices.

Recommended Readings

Alexander's Care of the Patient in Surgery. (2011, 14th ed.), Chapter 3: Infection prevention and control in the perioperative setting.

Perioperative Standards and Recommended Practices. (2013), Recommended practices:
- Selection and use of packaging systems for sterilization.
- Sterilization.

Berry and Kohn's Operating Room Technique. (2013, 12th ed.), Chapter 18: Sterilization.

Competency for Safe Patient Care During Operative and Invasive Procedures. (2009), Chapter 14: Monitor and control the environment.

Key Words

Biological indicator, Bowie-Dick air removal test, chemical indicator, pressure, temperature

Activity — Do You Know?

What is the image to the right?
What is its purpose?
How is it used?
Was the test successful or not?

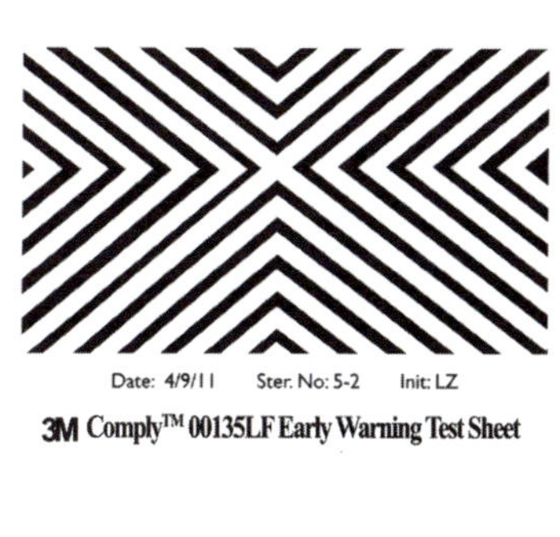

Activity — Matching

Match the indicator to its definition.

Class I _____   A. time, pressure, temperature readout

Class II _____   B. single-variable indicator

Class III _____   C. used to monitor every implant load

Class IV _____   D. used on outside of every package

Class V _____   E. Bowie-Dick

Physical monitor _____   F. multi-variable indicator

Biological indicator _____   G. reacts to all critical parameters

Activity — Critical Thinking

You are the circulator opening a set of instruments for an open reduction and internal fixation of a left ankle. There are three trays of specialty instrumentation, including implantable plates and screws for this procedure. All trays are labeled and identified with the same load number. All indicator tapes outside of the wrapped trays have turned color, indicating steam exposure. One of the trays does not have a chemical indicator inside of the tray. The other two have chemical indicators that have turned color, indicating effective steam penetration. The case is scheduled to begin in 30 minutes.

1. Can you assume that the instrumentation is sterile based on the two trays having positive indicators and being from the same cycle of the sterilizer?

2. What are your options? What are the pros and cons of each?

3. How could this situation be avoided in the future?

Additional Reading/Resources

Chard, R. (2009). Tracking sterilization loads that contain implants. *AORN Journal, 90*(1), 117.

Mitchell, S. (2009). Class 6 emulating chemical indicators and process challenge packs. *AORN Journal, 90*(2), 279-280.

Module 6: Safe Handling Practices for Hazardous and Biohazardous Materials

Introduction

Any substance that poses a health threat to people or the environment requires special care in both handling and disposition. Perioperative nurses are responsible for ensuring that the work environment is safe for patients, fellow workers, and themselves.

Competency Outcomes

To successfully complete the activities in this module, you will need to be able to:

1. Identify potential sources of injury to personnel in the perioperative setting.
2. Employ methods for maintaining a safe environment.

Recommended Readings

Alexander's Care of the Patient in Surgery. (2011, 14th ed.), Chapter 30: Workplace issues and staff safety.

Perioperative Standards and Recommended Practices. (2013), Recommended practices for safe environment of care.

Berry and Kohn's Operating Room Technique. (2013, 12th ed.), Chapter 13: Potential sources of injury to the caregiver and the patient.

Competency for Safe Patient Care During Operative and Invasive Procedures. (2009), Chapter 14: Monitor and control the environment.

Key Words

Bloodborne pathogen, hands-free zone, MSDS, neutral zone, sharps safety, standard precautions

Activity — Can You Top This?

List as many ways as possible to decrease the number of sharps injuries.

Activity — True or False

A smoke evacuation system is not needed for laparoscopic procedures.

TRUE   FALSE

Activity — Short Answer

What practices should be implemented for the safe use of methyl methacrylate bone cement?

Activity — Multiple Choice

What is the *best* way to dispose of unused chemotherapy agents?

A. Flush them down the hopper.

B. Place in impervious container and send with patient.

C. Follow federal, state, and local laws in consultation with health care organization's pharmacist.

D. Place them in a hazardous transport container and dispose of it with other OR waste.

E. Follow OSHA guidelines.

Additional Reading/Resources

Mellinger, E., Skinker, L., Sears, D., Gardner, D., et al. (2010). Safe handling of chemotherapy in the perioperative setting. *AORN Journal, 91*(4), 435-453.

National Institute for Occupational Safety and Health (NIOSH). (2004). Preventing occupational exposures to antineoplastic and other hazardous drugs in health care settings. NIOSH Alert (Pub no. 2004-165). Washington, DC.

Willemson-McBride, T.L. (2009). Safe handling of cytotoxic agents: A team approach. *AORN Journal, 90*(5), 731-740.

> **"Go To" Activity — Skill Building**
>
> Locate the MSDS reference in your department.
>
> Talk with your risk mitigation manager or infection prevention specialist about your facility's exposure control plan.

Chapter Summary

Sterility is the hallmark of the operating room; it is the one defining characteristic that makes the environment safe for surgery. Your knowledge and application of the principles and practice of disinfection and sterilization have a direct impact on patient safety. The disinfection and sterilization of instruments begin at the point of use — when a sterile instrument is delivered to the sterile field. Though we may not initially process the instruments and equipment, we are accountable to our patients for delivering the safest possible patient care.

Glossary

Airborne precautions — Precautions used when caring for patients with known or suspected microorganisms that can be transmitted by the airborne route.

Aseptic technique — Practices that restrict microorganisms in the environment and on equipment and supplies and that prevent normal body flora from contaminating the surgical wound.

Association for the Advancement of Medical Instrumentation (AAMI) — Alliance of health care professions dedicated to increasing the understanding, safety, and efficacy of medical instrumentation.

Bioburden — Amount of microbial load on an item before sterilization.

Biohazardous waste — Contaminated with blood, body fluids, or tissues capable of transmitting infection.

Biologic indicator — A sterilization process monitoring device containing a known population of highly resistant spores that is used to test the effectiveness of sterilization.

Chemical indicator — A device used to monitor the attainment of one or more critical parameters of the sterilization cycle. A characteristic color change indicates a defined level of exposure based on the conditions within the sterilization chamber.

Cleaning — Using friction, detergent, and water to remove soil and debris. Cleaning removes, rather than kills, microorganisms.

Contact precautions — Precautions designed to reduce the risk of transmission of infectious microorganisms transmitted by direct or indirect contact.

Critical item — Item that contacts the vascular system or enters sterile tissue or body cavities; poses the highest risk for transmission of infection.

Decontamination — Cleaning and disinfecting or sterilizing processes carried out to make contaminated items safe to handle.

Disinfection — The process of eliminating many or all pathogenic organisms except bacterial spores from inanimate objects.

Droplet precautions — Precautions used when caring for patients with known or suspected microorganisms that can be transmitted by infectious large particle (i.e., 5 microns or larger) droplets.

Enzymatic cleaner — Cleaning agent that uses enzymes to remove protein from surgical instruments.

Food and Drug Administration (FDA) — An agency of the U.S. Department of Health and Human Services, responsible for protecting and promoting public health through the regulation and supervision of medical devices.

Germicide — A disinfectant that kills pathogenic microorganisms.

Hazardous waste — Any substance that poses a health threat to persons or the environment.

High-level disinfection — Process that kills all microorganisms with the exception of high numbers of bacterial spores and prions. Inactivates *Mycobacterium tuberculosis*, Hepatitis B, HIV, vegetative bacteria, and some spores and fungi. It is not effective against prions that cause Creutzfeld-Jacob disease.

Immediate use sterilization (previously known as "flash" sterilization) — Sterilization of unwrapped items at point of use for a specific patient or procedure, using an abbreviated sterilization cycle.

Intermediate-level disinfection — Level of disinfection that kills *Mycobacterium tuberculosis*, vegetative bacteria, most viruses, and most fungi, but does not necessarily kill bacterial spores.

Loaner instrumentation — Borrowed or consigned surgical instruments, equipment, and supplies brought in from outside the facility.

Low-level disinfection — Level of disinfection that kills most bacteria, some viruses, and some fungi. It cannot be relied on to kill resistant organisms or spores.

Non-critical item — Item that comes in contact with intact skin but not with mucous membranes, sterile tissue, or the vascular system.

Pathogen — Any microorganism capable of causing disease.

Personal protective equipment (PPE) — Specialized equipment or supplies (gown, gloves, mask, eye protection, etc.) used to protect the worker from injury or exposure to environmental hazards.

Prion — Infectious protein particle responsible for transmissible spongiform encephalopathies (i.e., Creutzfeld-Jacob disease in humans).

Semi-critical item — Item that comes in contact with mucous membranes or non-intact skin.

Standard precautions — Precautions used in the care of all patients, regardless of known or suspected disease processes. As used in the Job Analysis, this term refers to the standard and transmission-based precautions policies and procedures as developed by the CDC and OSHA.

Sterilization — Process that kills all living microorganisms (bacteria, fungi, virus, and bacterial spores).

Surgical conscience/sterile conscience — Awareness that develops from a keen understanding of the importance of strict adherence to principles of aseptic technique.

Transmission-based precautions — Practices for patients with specific or suspected infectious processes with highly transmissible or epidemiologically important pathogens. Includes airborne, droplet, and contact precautions.

References

AORN. (2013). *Perioperative Standards and Recommended Practices*. Denver: AORN, Inc.

Occupational Safety and Health Administration (OSHA). (2002). *OSHA Safety Fact Sheet: Ethylene oxide.* Retrieved Feb. 7, 2013, from http://www.osha.gov/OshDoc/data_General_Facts/ethylene-oxide-factsheet.pdf

Phillips, N. (2013). *Berry and Kohn's Operating Room Technique* (12th ed.). St. Louis: Mosby.

Phippen, M.L., Ulmer, B.C., & Wells, M.P. (2009). *Competency for Safe Patient Care During Operative and Invasive Procedures.* Denver: CCI.

Rothrock, J.C. (Ed.). (2011). *Alexander's Care of the Patient in Surgery* (14th ed.). St. Louis: Mosby.

Answers to Chapter 6 Activities

Module 1: Microbiological considerations related to infection control principles — Pages 174-177

Activity — Fill in the Blank

The most important component of standard precautions is ***hand hygiene.***

Source: Rothrock, J.C. (Ed.). (2011). *Alexander's Care of the Patient in Surgery* (14th ed., p. 62). St. Louis: Mosby.

Activity — Short Answer

What nursing interventions should be implemented while caring for a patient with each of the following transmission-based precautions?

Contact:

Standard PPE (gloves, gown, mask, protective eye wear). Ensure precautions are maintained during patient transport; adequately clean/disinfect patient care equipment between patient uses. Consider using patient-dedicated equipment.

Airborne:

Standard PPE (gloves, gown, protective eye wear). In addition, health care personnel should

wear an OSHA-approved N-95 mask. Patients should wear a surgical mask during transport and be placed in an airborne isolation room or a room that is ventilated to the outside. If case can not be delayed until patient is no longer infectious, perform procedures at end of day when least number of patients/staff is present. Place a bacterial filter on endotracheal tube. Enforce strict traffic control. After case is completed, leave room closed for at least 28 minutes, until air in room has been completely exchanged. People entering room before that should wear N-95 mask and appropriate PPE.

Droplet:

Standard PPE (gloves, gown, protective eye wear). Mask must be worn within 3 feet of patient. Position patients at least 3 feet from other patients. Patients should wear surgical mask during transport. Adequately clean/disinfect patient care equipment between patient uses.

Source: AORN. (2013). Recommended practices: Prevention of transmissible infections, pp. 334-338. In *Perioperative Standards and Recommended practices*. Denver: AORN, Inc.

Activity — Stop the Spread

For each disease, choose the appropriate transmission based precautions and associated PPE.

Disease	Transmission-based precaution	PPE
Human immunodeficiency virus (HIV)	*Contact*	*Gloves, gown, mask, protective eye wear*
Mycobacterium tuberculosis	*Airborne*	*NIOSH-approved N-95 respirator*
Hepatitis B	*Contact*	*Gloves, gown, mask, protective eye wear.*
Staphylococcus aureus	*Contact*	*Gloves, gown, mask, protective eye wear.*
Clostridium difficile	*Contact*	*Gloves, gown, mask, protective eye wear.*
Pseudomonas	*Contact, droplet*	*Gloves, gown, protective eye wear. Mask when within 3 feet of person.*
Varicella	*Airborne*	*NIOSH-approved N-95 respirator unless demonstrates adequate immunity either by disease or immunization; if immune, surgical mask is adequate.*
Influenza	*Droplet*	*Mask when within 3 feet of person.*

Source: AORN. (2013). Recommended practices: Prevention of transmissible infections, pp. 334-338, 350. In *Perioperative Standards and Recommended Practices*. Denver: AORN, Inc.

Activity — True or False

Using an alcohol-based hand rub is the appropriate hand sanitizing method after caring for a patient with *Clostridium difficile.*

False. Hand washing after caring for a patient with Clostridium difficile must be done with antimicrobial soap and water.

Source: Rothrock, J.C. (Ed.). (2011). *Alexander's Care of the Patient in Surgery* (14th ed., p. 51). St. Louis: Mosby.

Activity — Critical Thinking

You have just cared for a patient who is suspected of having Creutzfeld-Jacob disease (CJD). What is the preferred method for inactivating prions on semi-critical and critical devices?

Gravity steam sterilization for 30 minutes at 131˚ C (268˚ F) or dynamic air removal steam sterilization for 18 minutes at 134˚ C to 138˚ C (273˚ F to 280˚ F).

Source: AORN. (2013). Recommended practices cleaning and care of surgical instruments and powered equipment, pp. 497-499. In *Perioperative Standards and Recommended Practices.* Denver: AORN, Inc.

Case Study Activity

In evaluating Mrs. M., what risk factors for a surgical site infection do you find?

Diabetes, obesity, smoker

Source: Phippen, M.L., Ulmer, B.C., & Wells, M.P. (2009). *Competency for Safe Patient Care During Operative and Invasive Procedures,* p. 292. Denver: CCI.

Module 2: Cleaning and disinfecting instruments and supplies — Pages 178-181

Activity — Multiple Choice

The most reliable source for information regarding processing of instruments and equipment is:
   A. OSHA regulations
   B. TJC requirements
   C. FDA protocols
   D. Manufacturers' instructions

D. Manufacturers' instructions

Source: AORN. (2013). Recommended practices cleaning and care of surgical instruments and powered equipment, p. 485. In *Perioperative Standards and Recommended Practices.* Denver: AORN, Inc.

Activity — Matching

Match the item to its definition

1. Non-critical - ***C***

A. Enters sterile tissues including the vascular system

2. Semi-critical - ***B***

B. Contacts non-intact skin and mucous membranes

3. Critical - ***A***

C. Contacts intact skin or does not come in contact with the patient

Source: AORN. (2013). Recommended practices for high-level disinfection, pp. 459-460. In *Perioperative Standards and Recommended Practices*. Denver: AORN, Inc.

Activity — Put It In Its Place

Match the following items to the potential for transmitting infection and their appropriate method of processing.

Disease transmission risk	Item	Method of processing
Non-critical	***Mayo stand***	Low-level disinfection
Non-critical	***Blood pressure cuff*** ***Tourniquet cuff*** ***Doppler***	Intermediate-level disinfection
Semi-critical	***Laryngoscope*** ***Colonoscope***	High-level disinfection
Critical	***Balfour retractor*** ***Urinary catheter***	Sterilization

Source: AORN. (2013). Recommended practices for high-level disinfection, p. 460. In *Perioperative Standards and Recommended Practices*. Denver: AORN.

Activity — Do You Know?

Check all of the following that represent proper management of instruments used during a surgical procedure:

A. ***No — Instruments should be kept clean during the procedure with sterile WATER. Saline can damage instruments over time.***

B. ***Correct***

C. ***Correct — Good communication with SPD enhances their ability to meet the needs of the OR.***

D. ***No — All instruments opened onto the sterile field are considered contaminated; keep sets together to facilitate SPD's ability to process and return complete sets to the OR.***

E. ***Correct — If instruments are returned to SPD immediately this may not be necessary. If***

instruments remain in the OR for a significant length of time, they should be soaked in an enzymatic cleaner. Instruments should be removed from the soak before transport to SPD; if transported in the enzymatic solution, the container must be sealed to prevent spillage.

Source: Rothrock, J.C. (Ed.). (2011). *Alexander's Care of the Patient in Surgery* (14th ed., pp. 68-69). St. Louis: Mosby.

Activity — Scramble

Number the following steps in high-level disinfection in the correct order:

5 - Flush lumens with disinfectant.
3 - Clean the instrument.
6 - Time the immersion cycle.
1 - Wear appropriate PPE.
9 - Document results of processing.
2 - Check solution for minimum effective concentration.
8 - Deliver to point of use without contaminating.
7 - Rinse with sterile water.
4 - Immerse instrument in disinfectant according to manufacturer's recommendations.

Source: AORN. (2013). Recommended practices for high-level disinfection, p. 463. In *Perioperative Standards and Recommended Practices*. Denver: AORN, Inc.

Activity — Short Answer

How long can an item that has been high-level disinfected be stored before use?

Items that are high-level disinfected must be used immediately.

Source: AORN. (2013). Recommended practices for high-level disinfection, p. 465. In *Perioperative Standards and Recommended Practices*. Denver: AORN, Inc.

Activity — Critical Thinking

A surgical instrumentation vendor arrives at 0715 for your scheduled 0730 anterior/posterior spinal fusion case with a set of implants that he states "are in the process of being FDA approved and the surgeon wants to trial." The implants have been sterilized at another facility and are covered with a heavy plastic dust cover. What is your response?

Loaner instrumentation should be examined, cleaned, and sterilized by the receiving health care organization before use. This case is not emergent, so immediate use sterilization should not be considered. In addition, the patient should be notified of the experimental nature of the implant and its benefits, risks, and alternatives, and should consent to its use. The ethics

committee of the facility should investigate this implant before approval for its use is granted. A policy should be in place for accepting and processing loaner instrumentation. The vendor must meet facility, state, and federal safety regulations.

Sources: AORN. (2013). Recommended practices for cleaning and care of instruments, p. 486; Guidance statement: Role of the health care industry representative, pp. 541-542. In *Perioperative Standards and Recommended Practices*. Denver: AORN, Inc.; Rothrock, J.C. (Ed.). (2011). *Alexander's Care of the Patient in Surgery* (14th ed, p. 45). St. Louis: Mosby.

Module 3: Packaging and sterilization of instruments and supplies — Pages 182-186

Activity — Fill in the Blank

Complete the chart for typical cycle times for *dynamic air removal (prevacuum)* steam sterilization.

Item	Exposure time at 270° F (132° C)	Minimum dry time	Exposure time at 275° F (135° C)	Minimum dry time
Wrapped instruments	*4 min.*	*20-30 min.*	*3 min.*	*16 min.*
Textile packs	*4 min.*	*5-20 min.*	*3 min.*	*3 min.*

Source: AORN. (2013). Recommended practices for sterilization. In *Perioperative Standards and Recommended Practices*, p. 519. Denver: AORN, Inc.

Complete the chart for typical cycle times for *gravity displacement* steam sterilization.

Item	Exposure time at 250° F (121° C)	Minimum dry time	Exposure time at 270° F (132° C)	Minimum dry time	Exposure time at 275° F (135° C)	Minimum dry time
Wrapped instruments	*30 min.*	*15-30 min.*	*15 min.*	*15-30 min.*	*NA*	*NA*
Textile packs	*30 min.*	*15 min.*	*25 min.*	*15 min.*	*10 min.*	*30 min.*

Source: AORN. (2013). Recommended practices for sterilization. In *Perioperative Standards and Recommended Practices*, p. 518. Denver: AORN, Inc.

Activity — Critical Thinking

Use the autoclave tape below to answer the following questions:

```
========================
=======PREVAC=======
========================
CYCLE   START   AT   10:53:06A
                ON      4/06/11

CYCLE   COUNT           28827
OPERATOR _______________________
   STERLIZER            VAC S2

        STER TEMP   =   270.0F
     CONTROL TEMP   =   273.0F
        STER TIME   =   4 MIN
        DRY TIME    =   0 MIN

                         V=inHg
-TIME               T=F  P=psig

C   10:53:06A   146.4    0P
C   10:54:05A   249.1    21P
C   10:55:19A   181.8    22V
C   10:55:39A   249.7    26P
C   10:56:59A   110.5    22V
C   10:57:15A   237.5    26P
C   10:58:31A   168.2    22V
C   10:58:46A   247.3    26P
C   11:00:02A   179.6    23V
S   11:00:40A   270.1    32P
S   11:02:40A   273.5    32P
E   11:04:40A   273.2    31P
E   11:04:55A   233.7    3P
E   11:04:56A   232.6    2P
Z   11:05:08A   207.3    0P

LOAD                    040602

     TEMP MAX  =  273.8F
     TEMP MIN  =  270.1F

CONDITION     = 7:34
STERILIZE     = 4:00
EXHAUST       = 0:29
TOTAL CYCLE   = 12:03

========================
=    READY TO UNLOAD    =
========================

* NOT READY         3:22:48P
DOOR UNLOCKED
```

1. What method of sterilization is this?
Dynamic air removal (prevacuum) steam sterilization, 4 minute cycle, immediate use

2. What type(s) of instruments can be processed using this method of sterilization?
Metal, porous, with lumens

3. What type(s) of monitoring should be used for this method of sterilization?
Class 5 chemical indicator with every load, plus a rapid-action biological indicator (BI) if implants are being sterilized (NOT recommended to sterilize implants using this method except in cases of emergency when no other option is available). The load should be quarantined until the results of the BI are available.

4. Under what set of circumstances should this method of sterilization be used?
Use of a rigid sterilization container designed for immediate-use sterilization; insufficient time to process by the preferred wrapped or container method. Items still must be properly decontaminated prior to sterilization. Packaging/wrappers/towels should not be used unless sterilizer is specifically designed for such. Items are to be used immediately.

5. When is it inappropriate to use this method of sterilization?
As a substitute for insufficient inventory; late arrival of loaner instrumentation and implantable devices; and when items will not be used immediately.

6. How should this cycle be documented?
Autoclave identification number, date, time, load number, type of sterilizer/cycle, contents of load, cycle parameters checked (e.g., temperature, duration of cycle), results of process monitoring indicators, operator, patient, and reason for immediate use sterilization.

Source: AORN. (2013). Recommended practices for sterilization. In *Perioperative Standards and Recommended Practices*, pp. 518-521, 532-533. Denver: AORN, Inc.

Activity — Short Answer

What is unique about packaging for hydrogen peroxide gas plasma sterilizers?

Hydrogen peroxide is incompatible with cellulose and will cause the load to abort; hence, no paper or linen can be used for packaging.

Source: Rothrock, J.C. (Ed.). (2011). *Alexander's Care of the Patient in Surgery* (14th ed., pp. 80-81). St. Louis: Mosby.

Activity — Fill in the Blank

1. The microorganism used in biologic indicators is ***Geobacillus stearothermophilus***.

   Source: AORN. (2013). Recommended practices for sterilization. In *Perioperative Standards and Recommended Practices*, p. 533. Denver: AORN, Inc.

2. A limitation for using low-temperature hydrogen peroxide gas plasma sterilization is ***length of instrument lumen***.

   Source: AORN. (2013). Recommended practices for sterilization. In *Perioperative Standards and Recommended Practices*, p. 524. Denver: AORN, Inc.

3. During sterilization of double paper-plastic pouch packages, the packages should be placed ***paper-to-paper.***

   Source: AORN. (2013). Recommended practices for packaging systems. In *Perioperative Standards and Recommended Practices*, p. 507. Denver: AORN, Inc.

4. Which of the following sterilization methods is NOT considered low-temperature?

Steam autoclave

   Source: Rothrock, J.C. (Ed.). (2011). *Alexander's Care of the Patient in Surgery* (14th ed., pp. 80, 81, 215). St. Louis: Mosby.

Module 4: Principles of transporting and storing sterile supplies — Pages 186-188

Activity — Know Your Numbers

Sterile items should be stored at least ***8-10*** inches above the floor, at least ***18*** inches below sprinkler heads, and at least ***2*** inches from outside walls.

   Source: AORN. (2013). Recommended practices for sterilization. In *Perioperative Standards and Recommended Practices*, p. 529. Denver: AORN, Inc.

Activity — Fill in the Blank

Shelf life of a packaged sterile item is ***event related.***

   Source: AORN. (2013). Recommended practices for sterilization. In *Perioperative Standards and Recommended Practices*, p. 529. Denver: AORN, Inc.

Activity — Multiple Choice

A flexible endoscope should be high-level disinfected before use if it has been unused for

C. five days.

Source: AORN. (2013). Recommended practices for cleaning and processing endoscopes. In *Perioperative Standards and Recommended Practices*, p. 478. Denver: AORN, Inc.

Activity — Critical Thinking

You send an orderly to pick up a pacemaker battery that has just been delivered to the receiving area of central services. The battery is in a sealed, sterile package and is still in its cardboard shipping carton. You are busy, so the orderly places the carton on a prep table inside the room. What action should be taken?

The shipping carton should be immediately removed from the sterile area. It is a reservoir for dust and other contaminants. The prep table should be disinfected with a hospital-grade germicide. The orderly should be instructed on the appropriate way to transport sterile supplies in the OR.

Source: AORN. (2013). Recommended practices for sterilization. In *Perioperative Standards and Recommended Practices*, p. 529. Denver: AORN, Inc.

Case Study Activity

Your scrub person has requested that you open the basic major pan for Mrs. M.'s case in anticipation of an open cholecystectomy. You bring in the wrapped pan of instruments and open it appropriately on a small table. As you remove the lid, you notice beads of water on the inside of the tray. The chemical indicator is present, and its color change indicates effective steam penetration. The tray was in its customary location in the sterile supply room.

1. Are the instruments sterile?

No. Wrapped instruments that are opened and found to be wet cannot be considered sterile.

2. What are your options?

The instruments should be replaced with new instrumentation. If immediate-use sterilization is necessary, the instruments should be decontaminated appropriately first.

3. What is the significance of the load cycle lot number in this instance?

The load cycle lot number will need to be tracked to recall all other items in that load for possible wetness and contamination. Autoclave failure and corrective action will need to be documented and reported to OR and SPD managers, infection prevention, and quality assurance. If the sterilizer has malfunctioned, surgeons will need to be contacted with patient information.

Source: AORN. (2013). Recommended practices for sterilization. In *Perioperative Standards and Recommended Practices*, pp. 509, 519, 531-533. Denver: AORN, Inc.

Module 5: Principles of biological and chemical monitoring — Pages 189-191

Activity — Do You Know?

What is the figure on the right? What is its purpose? How is it used? Was the test successful or not?

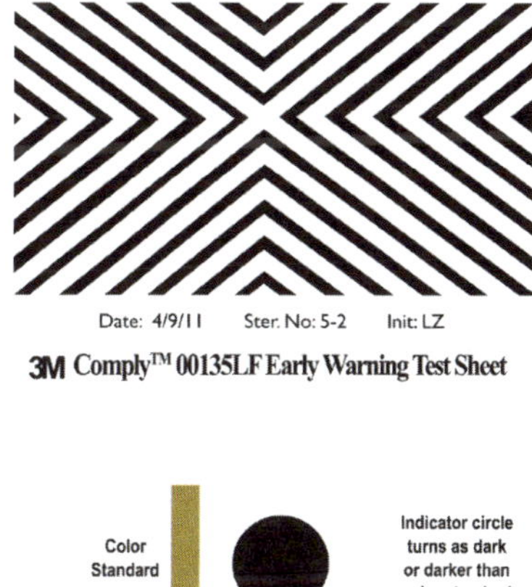

This is a chemical indicator Class 2 Bowie-Dick air removal test. It is used to detect residual air in the dynamic air-removal sterilizer. The graph is wrapped in the center of a test pack and placed on the lower shelf of an empty sterilizer chamber. The sterilizer is then run. It is used to measure the efficacy of the air removal system, not sterility. This test is a "pass."

Source: AORN. (2013). Recommended practices for sterilization. In *Perioperative Standards and Recommended Practices*, pp. 534-535, 537. Denver: AORN, Inc.

Activity — Matching

Match the indicator to its definition.

Class I - **D**	A. time, pressure, temperature readout
Class II - **E**	B. single-variable indicator
Class III - **B**	C. used to monitor every implant load
Class IV - **F**	D. used on outside of every package
Class V - **G**	E. Bowie-Dick
Physical monitor - **A**	F. multi-variable indicator
Biological indicator - **C**	G. reacts to all critical parameters

Source: AORN. (2013). Recommended practices for sterilization. In *Perioperative Standards and Recommended Practices*, pp. 534-535. Denver: AORN, Inc.

Activity — Critical Thinking

You are the circulator opening a set of instruments for an open reduction and internal fixation of a left ankle. There are three trays of specialty instrumentation, including implantable plates and screws for this procedure. All trays are labeled and identified with the same load number. All indicator tapes outside of the wrapped trays have turned color, indicating steam exposure. One of the trays does not have a chemical indicator inside of the tray. The other two have chemical indicators that have turned color, indicating effective steam penetration. The case is scheduled to begin in 30 minutes.

1. Can you assume that the instrumentation is sterile based on the two trays having positive indicators and being from the same cycle of the sterilizer?

You cannot assume that the instrumentation is sterile based on the results of the other trays from the same cycle of the same sterilizer. There is no definitive way to determine that steam reached the inner contents of the tray without an indicator.

2. What are your options? What are the pros and cons of each?

Is a sterile replacement tray available? If not, then the choices are:
- *Delaying the case may present an inconvenience to the patient and surgical team. However, appropriate processing of the instrumentation to provide sterile implants takes precedence and will help ensure optimal results for the patient.*
- *Immediate use (flash) sterilization is not recommended for any instrumentation, including implantable devices (e.g., plates and screws). If this option is chosen, a rapid-action biological indicator as well as a chemical indicator must be used, and the instruments must be quarantined until the results are read. The risk of contamination increases with flash sterilization because of the additional handling required to transport the tray from the sterilizer to the field.*

3. How could this situation be avoided in the future?

Planning and coordination will alleviate the need for flash sterilization. This includes scheduling cases appropriately (e.g., not scheduling cases requiring the same instrumentation back-to-back) and ensuring adequate numbers of instruments are available to perform multiple cases without flash sterilizing instruments. Notify sterile processing department of incident.

Source: AORN. (2013). Recommended practices for sterilization. In *Perioperative Standards and Recommended Practices*, p. 519-521, 531-533. Denver: AORN, Inc.

Module 6: Safe handling practices for hazardous and biohazardous materials — Pages 191-193

Activity — Can You Top This?

List as many ways as possible to decrease the number of sharps injuries.

Sample responses:
- *Use a neutral zone for passing sharps.*
- *Double glove.*
- *Use blunt suture needles.*
- *Fill the sharps container only ¾ full.*
- *Organize Mayo and back table so that sharp instruments are pointing away from the person setting up.*
- *Use a heavy clamp or needle holder, not fingers, to put scalpel blades on and off handle.*
- *Put sharp instruments (towel clips, rakes, etc.) in a separate container and notifying decontamination person.*
- *Keep hands away from surgical site when sharps are being used.*
- *Communicate when passing a sharp device.*

Source: Rothrock, J.C. (Ed.). (2011). *Alexander's Care of the Patient in Surgery* (14th ed., pp. 1263-1267). St. Louis: Mosby.

Activity — True or False

A smoke evacuation system is not needed for laparoscopic procedures. *FALSE*

Source: AORN. (2013). Recommended practices for minimally invasive surgery. p. 168. In *Perioperative Standards and Recommended Practices*. Denver: AORN, Inc.

Activity — Short Answer

What practices should be implemented for the safe use of methyl methacrylate bone cement?

- *Methods for reducing fumes (e.g., vacuum mixer, activated charcoal).*
- *Protective eyewear.*
- *Follow manufacturers' recommendations for mixing and required PPEs.*
- *Double glove.*
- *Use cement gun or mixing system to avoid contact with cement until it is the consistency of dough.*
- *Dispose of as a hazardous waste.*

Source: AORN. (2013). Recommended practices for a safe environment of care, pp. 231-233. In *Perioperative Standards and Recommended Practices*. Denver: AORN, Inc.

Activity — Multiple Choice

What is the best way to dispose of unused chemotherapy agents?

C. Follow federal, state, and local laws in consultation with health care organization's pharmacist.

Source: AORN. (2013). Recommended practices for a safe environment of care, p. 234; Recommended practices for medication safety, pp. 275-276. In *Perioperative Standards and Recommended Practices*. Denver: AORN, Inc.

NOTES

CHAPTER 7:
Emergency Situations

> **Test Specifications:**
> *8% of CNOR test questions are based on Emergency Situations.*

Introduction

The actions of the perioperative nurse in emergencies, regardless of the nature of the situation, are comparable to his or her responses during all patient care activities with the exception of time. There are two types of intraoperative emergencies: those which contributed to the need for the surgery, and those that emerge during the procedure itself.

Regardless of the nature of the emergency, the goals for treatment are:

1. Maintenance of an open airway.
2. Maintenance of circulating blood volume.
3. Perfusion of oxygen to vital organs to support function.

This chapter will help you review common emergencies and the appropriate nursing interventions necessary to successfully manage them. Anticipating and preventing emergencies by recognizing and treating early warning signs are emphasized.

Module 1: Anaphylaxis

Anaphylaxis is the most severe form of an allergic response because it involves many different body systems. Blood transfusion reactions and latex allergies are among the many adverse physiologic responses triggered by exposure to chemicals or drugs in the perioperative setting. Obtaining a thorough patient history of both medication and food allergies will help alert the perioperative nurse to possible adverse reactions and proactively address them.

Competency Outcomes

To successfully complete the activities in this module, you will need to be able to:

1. Describe the signs and symptoms of anaphylaxis.
2. Discuss nursing interventions for the patient experiencing an allergic reaction.

Recommended Readings

Alexander's Care of the Patient in Surgery. (2011, 14th ed.), pp. 40-42, 98, 1278-1280.

Perioperative Standards and Recommended Practices. (2013), Recommended practices for a safe environment of care.

Berry and Kohn's Operating Room Technique. (2013, 12th.), pp. 230-231, 248, 632.

Competency for Safe Patient Care During Operative and Invasive Procedures. (2009), pp. 96, 126-127, 158-160, 424-428.

Key Words

Allergy, anaphylactic shock, anaphylaxis, latex free, latex safe, sensitivity, transfusion reaction, type I IgE mediated response

Case Study Activity

Mrs. M.'s anesthesia care provider has determined that Mrs. M. is at high risk for developing a latex allergy. How will you prepare her operating room to decrease the risk for an allergic response to latex?

Activity — Do You Know?

Number the following interventions for a suspected blood transfusion reaction in the appropriate order.

___ Send a sample of the patient's urine to the lab.
___ Complete an occurrence/incident report.
___ Stop the transfusion.
___ Document and communicate reaction, interventions, and patient responses to the next caregiver.
___ Anticipate orders for emergency drugs.
___ Monitor the patient carefully.
___ Return unused blood, tubing, and a sample of the patient's blood to the blood bank.
___ Replace IV tubing and hang 0.9% sodium chloride.
___ Report reaction to surgeon and blood bank.

Activity — Critical Thinking

Many of the signs and symptoms of a blood transfusion reaction (e.g., chills, backache, shivering) are masked by a general anesthetic. How could you tell if your patient under a general anesthetic is having an adverse reaction to a blood transfusion?

Additional Reading/Resources

Briesemeister, E., & Burlingame, B.L. (2006). Shellfish and iodine allergies. *AORN Journal, 83*(2), 479.

Bundesen, I-M. (2008). Natural rubber latex: A matter of concern for nurses. *AORN Journal, 88*(2), 197-210.

Nelson, J. (2009). Latex in the perioperative setting: Strategies for patient and staff member safety. *AORN Journal, 89*(6), 1152.

> ### "Go To" Activity — Skill Building
>
> Ask your blood bank director to provide an in-service to your department on how blood products are processed and provided safely to patients.
>
> Review product selection guidelines for your facility and suggest that latex-free items be given priority in purchasing decisions.
>
> Review your department's policy and procedure related to safe blood transfusion practices.

Module 2: Cardiovascular Emergencies

Cardiac emergencies may arise from respiratory insufficiency or arrest, such as that seen in inadequate ventilation or hypoxia; complications related to the surgical intervention, such as blood loss, hypotension, or shock; or as a response to a disease process that has been exacerbated by the stress of surgery. Basic and advanced life-support skills must be implemented very quickly to help ensure a positive outcome for the patient.

Competency Outcomes

To successfully complete the activities in this module, you will need to be able to:

1. Identify common intraoperative cardiac emergencies.
2. Choose appropriate nursing interventions in managing the patient in cardiac arrest.

Recommended Readings

Alexander's Care of the Patient in Surgery. (2011, 14th ed.), pp. 272-275, 369; Chapter 23: Vascular surgery; Chapter 24: Cardiac surgery.

Berry and Kohn's Operating Room Technique. (2013, 12th ed.), Chapter 31: Potential perioperative complications (pp. 611-624).

Competency for Safe Patient Care During Operative and Invasive Procedures. (2009), pp. 158-160, 627.

Key Words

Advanced cardiac life support, autologous blood, blood loss, cardiac arrest, cardiopulmonary resuscitation, circulating blood volume, circulation, deep vein thrombosis, dysrhythmia, embolus, fluid replacement, hemorrhage, hypertension, hypotension, shock, thrombus, transfusion

> ### "Go To" Activity — Check It Out!
>
> Go to Question #36, DIC, under the Perioperative question of the week tab on your CD for another critical-thinking activity.

Activity — Critical Thinking

You are the scrub person for a patient scheduled for a craniotomy. The patient is in Fowler's position. As the bone flap is being elevated, the anesthesia care provider announces that she has diagnosed an air embolism. What is your first action?

Activity — Short Answer

You are monitoring an 83-year-old man who is having a lesion removed from his back under local anesthetic. His pulse and respirations are being assessed manually. He is in the prone position. He complains of shortness of breath, and then chest pain. What actions should be initiated?

Additional Reading/Resources

Allen, G. (2007). Cell saver blood transfusions. *AORN Journal, 85*(4), 823-824.

Allen, G. (2007). Reducing allogeneic transfusions. *AORN Journal, 85*(3), 640-642.

AORN. (2008). What was in those platelets? *AORN Journal, 92*(5), 598.

Babb, M. (2009). Clinical risk assessment: Identifying patients at high risk for heart failure. *AORN Journal, 89*(2), 273-288.

Dobbenga-Rhodes, Y.A. (2009). Responding to amniotic fluid embolism. *AORN Journal, 89*(6), 1079-1092.

Fisher, L. (2011). Perioperative care of the patient with sickle cell disease. *AORN Journal, 93*(1), 150-159.

John, T., Rodeman, R., & Colvin, R. (2008). Blood conservation in a congenital cardiac surgery program. *AORN Journal, 87*(6), 1180-1190.

Samudrala, S. (2008). Topical hemostatic agents in surgery: A surgeon's perspective. *AORN Journal, 88*(3), S2-S11.

> ## "Go To" Activity — Skill Building
>
> Enroll in an EKG course offered by your facility or community college, or an on-line program.
>
> Review the contents of your department's CODE or COR cart. Are age-appropriate supplies available based on your patient population?
>
> Set up and participate in a mock COR for your department.

Module 3: Respiratory Complications

The first priority in any emergency is to obtain and maintain a patent airway. Assisting the anesthesia care provider takes priority over any other nursing duties.

Competency Outcomes

To successfully complete the activities in this module, you will need to be able to:

1. Identify common respiratory emergencies.
2. Apply appropriate nursing interventions to manage respiratory emergencies.

Recommended Readings

Alexander's Care of the Patient in Surgery. (2011, 14th ed.), pp. 272, 278-280.

Perioperative Standards and Recommended Practices. (2013), Recommended practices for managing the patient receiving moderate sedation/analgesia.

Berry and Kohn's Operating Room Technique. (2013, 12th ed.), Chapter 31: Potential perioperative complications (pp. 608-611).

Competency for Safe Patient Care During Operative and Invasive Procedures. (2009), pp. 160-163, 626-627.

Key Words

Airway obstruction, anoxia, arterial blood gas, aspiration, atelectasis, bronchospasm, difficult airway, hypoxia, laryngospasm, pneumothorax, pulmonary edema, pulmonary embolism

Activity — Fill in the Blank

The first action in treating laryngospasm is to ___________________________ .

Activity — True or False

The purpose of a chest tube is to restore positive pressure in the intrapleural space.

TRUE   FALSE

"Go To" Activity — Check It Out!

Go to Question #22 under the Perioperative question of the week tab on your CD for an additional critical-thinking question.

Additional Reading/Resources

Allen, G. (2006). Anesthetic adverse events. *AORN Journal, 84*(6), 1067-1068.

AORN. (2008). Unexplained apnea during surgery. *AORN Journal, 87*(6), 1216, 1218.

Gazarian, P.K. (2006). Identifying risk factors for postoperative pulmonary complications. *AORN Journal, 84*(4), 615-625.

Module 4: Fire

OR fires are listed as "sentinel events." An oxygen-rich environment, flammable preps and drapes, and a plethora of ignition sources make the OR an especially high-risk area.

OR fires that involve the airway are some of the most devastating fires that involve patients. Laser and electrosurgical precautions must be implemented to prevent surgical fires of the airway.

Competency Outcomes

To successfully complete the activities in this module, you will need to be able to:

1. Identify steps to minimize the risk of fire.
2. Describe interventions to control a fire in the OR.

Recommended Readings

Alexander's Care of the Patient in Surgery. (2011, 14th ed.), pp. 32-33, 104, 235-237, 673.

Perioperative Standards and Recommended Practices. (2013), pp. 128-129, 146, 149-152, 220-224.

Berry and Kohn's Operating Room Technique. (2013, 12th ed.), pp. 224-226.

Competency for Safe Patient Care During Operative and Invasive Procedures. (2009), pp. 408-415.

Key Words

Burn, explosion, flammable, fuel, ignition source, oxygen, RACE, PASS

Activity — Critical Thinking

Toby, a 28-year-old male, has been admitted to the hospital for elective tonsillectomy/adenoidectomy. He has long hair, which he wears in a pony tail, and a medium length curly beard, trimmed neatly. He is healthy and in good physical shape. He has decided to have this surgery because of the snoring his wife complains about nightly, and the frequent sore throats, which have become annoying. He is a non-smoker. His preoperative assessment reveals nothing remarkable. He takes only occasional ibuprofen or acetaminophen for sore muscles or a headache, a multivitamin, and no prescription meds. He has no known drug allergies. He is 5' 8" and weighs 175 lbs.

Toby is wheeled to the operating room and positioned supine with a foam donut under his head. He is intubated with a cuffed ET tube. The surgery is to be performed with a CO_2 laser and a tonsil tip electrocautery handpiece. The only prep performed is an antiseptic mouthwash swish.

As the surgeon uses the laser for the first time there is a flash of light and suddenly the patient's beard is smoking. Then the surgical drape catches fire!

What are your first actions?

What could you have done to prevent this fire?

Additional Reading/Resources

AORN. (2007). Fire safety in perioperative settings. *AORN Journal, 86*(Supplement 1), S141-S145.

Briesemeister, E., & Burlingame, B.L. (2006). Fires caused by hair gel. *AORN Journal, 83*(2), 479.

Seltzer, J. A. (2010). Flammable prep agents. *AORN Journal, 92*(1), 6.

Watson, D.S. (2010). New recommendations for prevention of surgical fires. *AORN Journal, 91*(4), 463-469.

Watson, D.S. (2009). Surgical fires: 100% preventable, still a problem. *AORN Journal, 90*(4), 589-593.

"Go To" Activity — Skill Building

Locate the gas shut-off valves, fire extinguishers, and evacuation routes in your department.

Review your facility's policy and procedure related to fire safety. Compare it to AORN's policy and procedure on fire safety in *Perioperative Standards and Recommended Practices*.

Ask your local fire department to provide an in-service on fire evacuation methods and use of fire extinguishers.

Participate in fire drills in your facility.

Module 5: Malignant Hyperthermia

Malignant hyperthermia (MH) is a potentially fatal complication of general anesthesia that requires immediate action by the surgical team. Even though it does not occur frequently, the perioperative nurse should be prepared for an MH crisis. Because the condition has a genetic component, all surgical patients should be screened for a family history of MH.

Competency Outcomes

To successfully complete the activities in this module, you will need to be able to:

1.   Identify triggering agents that will activate malignant hyperthermia.
2.   Recognize signs and symptoms of an impending MH crisis.

Recommended Readings

Alexander's Care of the Patient in Surgery. (2011, 14th ed.), pp. 128, 139-141, 276-277, 1093-1094.

Berry and Kohn's Operating Room Technique. (2013, 12th ed.), pp. 636-639.

Competency for Safe Patient Care During Operative and Invasive Procedures. (2009), pp. 163-164.

Key Words

Acidosis, calcium, Dantrium, dantrolene sodium, dysrhythmia, hypercarbia, hyper-kalemia, hypermetabolic, hyperthermia, tachycardia, trigger

Activity — Do You Know?
Circle the agents known to trigger malignant hyperthermia:

Barbiturates	Ketamine
Benzodiazepines	Lidocaine
Bupivacaine	Morpine sulfate
Dantrolene sodium	Nitrous oxide
Desflurane	Pancuronium
Enflurane	Propofol
Halothane	Sevoflurane
Isoflurane	Succinylcholine

Activity — Critical Thinking

Which of the following is an early sign of malignant hyperthermia?

Elevated temperature   Hyperglycemia   Metabolic acidosis   Tachycardia

Activity — Patient Scenario

Mr. J., a 70-year-old male, comes to your hospital for a right total knee replacement. His past medical history includes a left inguinal hernia repair 20 years ago. He experienced no difficulties with anesthesia at that time. Significant history includes mild chronic obstructive lung disease and hypertension. He has smoked a pipe for the past 40 years and enjoys 1-2 mixed drinks several times a week. He is retired and considers himself in general good health. He has no known allergies. His current medications include lisinopril 12/25 once a day, a multi-vitamin, a maintenance inhaler, a nasal spray for his allergies, and one aspirin a day. The anesthesia care provider states his ASA score is 2. A rapid sequence induction is planned, because the patient had water with his medications this morning.

Mr. J. is transported to the OR suite at 0930. He is anesthetized, positioned, prepped, and draped. The surgical checklist is completed, including the time-out, with no issues identified. The surgery begins without incident.

At the same time that the knee prosthesis package is opened and the bone cement delivered to the field and mixed (1100), Mr. J.'s heart rate climbs to 120. The anesthesia care provider notes the patient is requiring more oxygen to maintain a normal oxygen saturation level. The circulating nurse notes that Mr. J.'s skin is becoming mottled with purple splotches. When the anesthesia care provider checks the placement of the endotracheal tube, she notes the jaw muscles are very tight. Mr. J.'s temperature is normal at 36.5° C.

1.   Highlight the signs in the scenario indicative of MH.

2.   What other conditions might you suspect?

Additional Reading/Resources

Denholm, B. (2007). Malignant hyperthermia. *AORN Journal, 85*(2), 403-408.

Hommertzheim, R., & Steinke, E.E. (2006). Malignant hyperthermia: The perioperative nurse's role. *AORN Journal, 83*(1), 149-164.

Malignant Hyperthermia Association of the United States (MHAUS). Healthcare professionals home page. Retrieved Feb. 27, 2013, from http://www.mhaus.org/healthcare-professionals/

> **"Go To" Activity — Check It Out!**
>
> Go to Question #7 under the Perioperative question of the week tab on your CD for an additional critical-thinking question.

Module 6: Trauma

Trauma care abides by the "golden hour" rule — the time immediately after an injury when interventions are likely to be most successful in achieving optimal outcomes. Nowhere is multidisciplinary collaboration more necessary than in providing care to the critically injured patient.

Competency Outcomes

To successfully complete the activities in this module, you will need to be able to:

1. Anticipate patient's physiologic and emotional response to the mechanism of injury.
2. Select nursing interventions based on prioritization of patient needs.

Recommended Readings

Alexander's Care of the Patient in Surgery. (2011, 14th ed.), Chapter 25: Pediatric surgery, pp. 1141-1145; Chapter 27: Trauma surgery.

Berry and Kohn's Operating Room Technique. (2013, 12th ed.), pp. 85, 126, 513, 575-576, 626-635, 682-683, 733, 744, 765, 800-801, 815-816, 919-920.

Competency for Patient Care During Operative and Invasive Procedures. (2009), Chapter 32: Trauma care.

Key Words

Acute respiratory distress syndrome, blunt trauma, dissociated intravascular coagulation (DIC), do-not-resuscitate (DNR), end of life care, mechanism of injury, multisystem, organ donor, rapid sequence intubation, trauma

Activity — Critical Thinking

You work in a rural community hospital that provides care to the surrounding ranching community. The hospital has 22 beds, one OR, and a labor deck. Cesarean sections are performed in the main OR. The majority of your surgical population is adults. Two surgeons who are on staff perform general, orthopedic, and gynecologic surgeries. A neurosurgeon, Dr. H., comes in once a month from a major teaching facility and performs lumbar discectomies. An ENT surgeon from the neighboring county's hospital has a weekly schedule of tonsillectomies and myringotomies, which are performed on an outpatient basis. A certified registered nurse anesthetist (CRNA) is the primary anesthesia care provider.

You have completed your schedule for the day, including two lumbar discectomies with Dr. H., when the emergency department (ED) pages you stat. It is 1930 on a Friday evening. When you and Dr. H. arrive, you find the staff busy caring for the victims of a multi-car accident involving three people. The driver of one car managed to walk to a farmhouse to call for help. His injuries include a broken left clavicle and a contusion over his left eye. The driver of the other car is alert and oriented.

Her vital signs are:

      Pulse: 120 bpm
      Respirations: 20/min
      Blood pressure: 96/50 mmHg
      Pulse oximeter: 92% on $2L/O_2$
      Temperature: 36.5° C

She is guarding her right abdomen, which is rigid. She has an IV of 0.9% normal saline infusing through a 16 ga intravenous catheter in her right antecubital. A CBC has been sent to the lab. The ED doctor suspects intra-abdominal bleeding.

This patient's primary concern, however, is for her 9-year-old son. He was sleeping in the back seat, not wearing a seat belt, and was ejected from the vehicle. When emergency medical technicians arrived, the child was unresponsive with shallow respirations of 10/minute. He was intubated at the scene. Fluids are being administered through a left tibial intraosseous infusion. Moistened 4X4 sponges have been placed over an open head wound. The child responds with decerebrate posturing to painful stimuli. When Dr. H. removes the sponges, meninges are visible.

The child's vital signs are:

      Pulse: 120 bpm
      Respirations: Ventilated via bag-valve mask at 18 breaths/minute
      Blood pressure: Palpated at 48 mm Hg
      Pulse oximeter: 90%
      Temperature: 34.8° C
      Glasgow coma scale: 5

Based on your available resources, discuss your plan of care for these patients.

Activity — Word Scramble

Find and circle the words from the list below. Words may be horizontal, vertical, or diagonal.

Perioperative Trauma Nursing

```
D N E O T T S T A B B I N G S
P U O C A R T N O C P U O C Y
D N D I N O I T A R T E N E P
I O E T T V J C R U S H I N G
S I C B A A E F O F E W D O Y
A S E U S G R P A G G Z U I T
S O L L S E Y E A L L K G S I
T L E L E T C I L A L U T I C
E P R E S O R R R E N S X C O
R X A T S T Y U O S C T Z E L
S E T S M Y T Z H F U C J D E
T R I F E A Q O C P H T A G V
I M O W N C T E C N A R T N E
X P N S T F Y R U J N I B D T
E R U P T U R E J Z W A X X G
```

ACCELERATION	NATURAL
ASSESSMENT	PENETRATION
BULLETS	RUPTURE
COUPCONTRACOUP	STABBINGS
CRUSHING	TAG
DECELERATION	TOE
DECISION	TRIAGE
DISASTERS	VELOCITY
ENTRANCE	
EXIT	
EXPLOSION	
FALLS	
FORCES	
GUNSHOT	
INJURY	

<table>
<tr><td>

**"Go To" Activity —
Check It Out!**

Go to Question #12 under the Perioperative question of the week tab on your CD for an additional critical-thinking question.

</td></tr>
</table>

Additional Reading/Resources

Anderson, M., & Leflore, J. (2008). Playing it safe: Simulated team training in the OR. *AORN Journal, 87*(4), 772-779.

Inoue, K. (2010). Caring for the perioperative patient with increased intracranial pressure. *AORN Journal, 91*(4), 511-518.

McArthur, B.J. (2006). Damage control surgery for the patient who has experienced multiple traumatic injuries. *AORN Journal, 84*(6), 991-1000.

Murdock, D.B. (2008). When there's no time to count. *AORN Journal, 87*(2), 322-323.

Neveleff, D.J, Kraiss, L.W., & Schulman, C.S. (2010). Implementing methods to improve perioperative hemostasis in the surgical and trauma settings. *AORN Journal, 92*(5), S1-S15.

Sakorafas, G.H., Tsiotou, A., Pananaki, M., & Peros, G. (2007). The role of surgery in the management of septic shock: Intra-abdominal causes of sepsis. *AORN Journal, 85*(2), 280-294.

Wright, I. (2007). Cerebral aneurysm: Treatment and perioperative nursing care. *AORN Journal, 85*(6), 1172-1186.

Module 7: Disasters

A disaster can be loosely defined as an event that overwhelms available resources. The event will dictate the type of response needed. Perioperative personnel may be mobilized more for their general nursing skills than their perioperative expertise.

Recommended Readings

Alexander's Care of the Patient in Surgery. (2011, 14th ed.), pp. 64-66.

Perioperative Standards and Recommended Practices. (2013), Recommended practices: Prevention of transmissible infections.

Berry and Kohn's Operating Room Technique. (2013, 12th ed.), pp. 20-21, 251.

Competency Outcomes

To successfully complete the activities in this module, you will need to be able to:

1. Review transmission routes for common bioterrorism agents.
2. Compare The Joint Commission's requirements for emergency preparedness with your facility's disaster plan.

"Go To" Activity — Check It Out!

Go to Question #50, Emergency situation, under the Perioperative question of the week tab on your CD for another critical-thinking activity.

Key Words

Bioterroism, bomb, mass casualty, natural disaster, preparedness, terrorism

Activity — Matching

Match the bioterrorism agent to its modes of transmission. Answers may be used more than once.

Anthrax _______	A. direct contact	E. aerosol
Smallpox _______	B. indirect contact	F. infected animal tissue
Plague _______	C. droplet	G. contaminated food or water
Tularemia _______	D. flea or rodent bite	H. arthropod bite
Botulism _______		

Additional Reading/Resources

Blanchard, J. (2006). Biological microorganism use in terrorism. *AORN Journal, 83*(3), 727.

Centers for Disease Control and Prevention. Bioterrorism. Retrieved Feb. 27, 2013, from http://emergency.cdc.gov/bioterrorism/

Centers for Disease Control and Prevention. Emergency preparedness and response: Mass casualty event preparedness and response. Retrieved March 1, 2013 from http://www.bt.cdc.gov/masscasualties/

Centers for Disease Control and Prevention. Mass casualties predictor. Retrieved Feb. 27, 2013, from http://www.bt.cdc.gov/masscasualties/predictor.asp

PBS Nova online (2009). History of biowarfare. Retrieved Feb. 27, 2013, from http://www.pbs.org/wgbh/nova/military/history-biowarfare.html (Note: Available as an interactive video and in print)

"Go To" Activity — Skill Building

Review your facility's emergency preparedness plan. Are The Joint Commission's requirements for mitigation, preparedness, response, and recovery incorporated?

Offer to update your department's telephone triage list.

Volunteer to serve as a resource for your local Red Cross or community health department.

Chapter Summary

One of the perioperative nurse's most important roles is that of patient advocate. In this role, the nurse must be prepared for any type of emergency that may occur in the surgical practice setting. Teamwork is important in achieving desired outcomes, but it takes on greater significance in an emergency. The perioperative nurse is in the unique role of coordinating the team effort and assisting other team members in appropriately preparing for and responding to an emergency in the OR.

Glossary

Activity — It's Your Turn

Using your resources, define the following terms found in this chapter.

Acid/base —

Anaphylaxis —

Anoxia —

Arterial blood gas —

Aspiration —

Atelectasis —

Cricoid pressure —

Difficult airway —

Embolus —

Hypercarbia —

Hypoxia —

Laryngospasm —

Latex free —

Latex safe —

Pneumothorax —

Pulmonary edema —

Pulmonary embolism —

Pulmonary hypertension —

Rapid sequence intubation —

Thrombus —

References

AORN. (2013). *Perioperative Standards and Recommended Practices*. Denver: AORN, Inc.

The Joint Commission. (2013). *Comprehensive Accreditation Manual for Hospitals: The Official Handbook* (Emergency Management). Oakbrook Terrace, IL: The Joint Commission.

Phillips, N. (2013). *Berry and Kohn's Operating Room Technique* (12th ed.). St. Louis: Mosby.

Phippen, M.L., Ulmer, B., & Wells, M.P. (2009). *Competencies for Safe Patient Care During Operative and Invasive Procedures*. Denver: CCI.

Rothrock, J.C. (Ed.). (2011). *Alexander's Care of the Patient in Surgery* (14th ed.). St. Louis: Mosby.

Simunek, L.C.A. (1996). Legal and ethical dimensions of perioperative practice. In S.S. Fairchild (Ed.), *Perioperative Nursing: Principles and Practice* (pp. 378-404). Philadelphia: Little, Brown and Company.

Sword, S.L.H. (1996). Organizational structure: The team concept. In S.S. Fairchild (Ed.), *Perioperative Nursing: Principles and Practice* (pp. 24-32). Philadelphia: Little, Brown and Company.

U.S. Department of Labor, Occupational Safety and Health Administration (OSHA). Hazard communication. Retrieved March 1, 2013, from http://www.osha.gov/dsg/hazcom/index.html

U.S. Office of Personnel Management (OPM). (1999). Patients' Bill of Rights. Retrieved Feb. 27, 2013, from http://www.opm.gov/healthcare-insurance/healthcare/reference-materials/#url=Bill-of-Rights

Answers to Chapter 7 Activities

Module 1: Anaphylaxis — Pages 209-211

Case Study Activity

Mrs. M.'s anesthesia care provider has determined that Mrs. M. is at high risk for developing a latex allergy. How will you prepare her operating room to decrease the risk for an allergic response to latex?

Responses may vary but should contain the following key components:

The goal is to provide a latex safe environment. Mrs. M.'s procedure is scheduled as the first case of the day, which will help reduce her exposure to airborne aerosolized latex. All products containing latex should be removed from the room (gloves, catheters, etc.). Medications should be delivered via a latex-free route. Non-latex gloves should be available. All supplies for the surgical procedure should be inspected, and latex-free items should be substituted if at all possible; if not possible, the surgeon and anesthesia care provider should be notified. If it is unclear whether an item contains latex, the manufacturer should be contacted. If the facility has a latex-free cart, it should be brought to the room. Double check that any item added to the sterile field is latex-free.

Equipment and medications should be available for treating an anaphylactic response if necessary. Mrs. M.'s latex allergy should be documented and communicated to other care providers. Latex precautions signs should be placed on the OR door and her transport bed. Traffic should be restricted in and out of the room.

Latex-free IV tubing should be used, or replace injection ports with 3-way stopcocks. Tape over any unused ports. If latex-free blood pressure cuffs are not available, wrap Mrs. M.'s arm with latex-free material to prevent contact of the cuff with her skin. Consider designating a patient-specific cuff to decrease the chances of using a latex cuff. Latex-containing drains (e.g., Penrose) should not be used.

Many facilities have incorporated a special latex allergy identification bracelet as part of their protocol. Mrs. M. should be counseled to notify all health care providers in the future as to her latex allergy status.

Source: AORN. (2013). Recommended practices for safe environment of care, pp. 229-231. In *Perioperative Standards and Recommended Practices*. Denver: AORN.

Activity — Do You Know?

Number the following interventions for a suspected blood transfusion reaction in the appropriate order.

6 - Send a sample of the patient's urine to the lab.
9 - Complete an occurrence/incident report.

1 - Stop the transfusion.

8 - Document and communicate reaction, interventions, and patient responses to next caregiver.

4 - Anticipate orders for emergency drugs.

7 - Monitor the patient carefully.

5 - Return unused blood, tubing, and a sample of the patient's blood to the blood bank.

2 - Replace IV tubing and hang 0.9% sodium chloride.

3 - Report reaction to surgeon and blood bank.

Source: Rothrock, J.C. (Ed.). (2011). *Alexander's Care of the Patient in Surgery* (14th ed., p. 41). St. Louis: Mosby.

Activity — Critical Thinking

Many of the signs and symptoms of a blood transfusion reaction (e.g., chills, backache, shivering) are masked by a general anesthetic. How could you tell if your patient under a general anesthetic is having an adverse reaction to a blood transfusion?

Signs may include blood in the urine, decreased or no urine output, hypotension, hyperthermia, or excessive or unusual bleeding.

Sources: Rothrock, J.C. (Ed.). (2011). *Alexander's Care of the Patient in Surgery* (14th ed., p. 41). St. Louis: Mosby; Phippen, M.L., Ulmer, B., & Wells, M.P. (2009). *Competencies for Safe Patient Care During Operative and Invasive Procedures,* p. 160. Denver: CCI.

Module 2: Cardiovascular emergencies — Pages 212-213

Activity — Critical Thinking

You are the scrub person for a patient scheduled for a craniotomy. The patient is in Fowler's position. As the bone flap is being elevated, the anesthesia care provider announces that she has diagnosed an air embolism. What is your first action?

Place bone wax over the exposed bone to seal it.

Source: Rothrock, J.C. (Ed.). (2011). *Alexander's Care of the Patient in Surgery* (14th ed., p. 168). St. Louis: Mosby.

Activity — Short Answer

You are monitoring an 83-year-old man who is having a lesion removed from his back under local anesthetic. His pulse and respirations are being assessed manually. He is in the prone position. He complains of shortness of breath, and then chest pain. What actions should be initiated?

Responses may vary but should include the following points:

The surgeon needs to be notified immediately and the surgery terminated. The patient should be returned to a position of comfort in the supine position. Additional assistance should be obtained (e.g., anesthesia care provider, manager, other staff members, the rapid response team,

CODE team, 911, etc.). Oxygen should be started per nasal cannula and additional monitoring (blood pressure, EKG, pulse oximeter) should be initiated. An IV line should be started. The CODE or COR cart should be brought to the room. The patient's cardiac history and current medications and allergies should be reviewed.

Source: AORN. (2013). Recommended practices for managing the patient receiving local anesthesia, pp. 410-411. In *Perioperative Standards and Recommended Practices*. Denver: AORN, Inc.

Module 3: Respiratory complications — Pages 213-214

Activity — Fill in the Blank

The first action in treating laryngospasm is to ***remove the irritating stimulus.***

Source: Rothrock, J.C. (Ed.). (2011). *Alexander's Care of the Patient in Surgery* (14th ed., p. 272). St. Louis: Mosby.

Activity — True or False

The purpose of a chest tube is to restore positive pressure in the intrapleural space. ***False.***

Source: Rothrock, J.C. (Ed.). (2011). *Alexander's Care of the Patient in Surgery* (14th ed., p. 946). St. Louis: Mosby.

Module 4: Fire — Pages 215-216

Activity — Critical Thinking

Toby, a 28-year-old male, has been admitted to the hospital for elective tonsillectomy/adenoidectomy. He has long hair, which he wears in a pony tail, and a medium length curly beard, trimmed neatly. He is healthy and in good physical shape. He has decided to have this surgery because of the snoring his wife complains about nightly, and the frequent sore throats, which have become annoying. He is a non-smoker. His preoperative assessment reveals nothing remarkable. He takes only occasional ibuprofen or acetaminophen for sore muscles or a headache, a multivitamin, and no prescription meds. He has no known drug allergies. He is 5' 8" and weighs 175 lbs.

Toby is wheeled to the operating room and positioned supine with a foam donut under his head. He is intubated with a cuffed ET tube. The surgery is to be performed with a CO_2 laser and a tonsil tip electrocautery handpiece. The only prep performed is an antiseptic mouthwash swish.

As the surgeon uses the laser for the first time there is a flash of light and suddenly the patient's beard is smoking. Then the surgical drape catches fire!

What are your first actions?

- ***Communicate the presence of the fire to all team members.***
- ***Pour saline or water slowly on the patient in the area of the fire.***
- ***Remove the surgical drapes.***

- ***Consult with the anesthesia care provider on necessary actions to extinguish an airway fire.***
- ***Assist the anesthesia care provider with disconnecting and removing the airway circuit.***
- ***Turn off the flow of oxygen.***
- ***Remove the ET tube.***
- ***Pour saline into the airway if instructed.***
- ***Re-establish the airway.***
- ***Call for help.***
- ***Notify the team leader or charge nurse.***
- ***Get a fire extinguisher if needed for surrounding area.***

Source: AORN. (2013). Recommended practices for laser safety, pp. 150, 152; Recommended practices for safe environment of care, pp. 222-223. In *Perioperative Standards and Recommended Practices*. Denver: AORN, Inc.

What could you have done to prevent this fire?

Coat facial hair with a water based gel and drape Toby with damp towels to further reduce flammability. The ET tube should be laser safe, and the cuff should be filled with saline and dye. Laser instruments (e.g., retractors and suctions) should be non-reflective. ESU handpiece tips should be coated with rubber or a non-reflective material from the manufacturer. Drapes should not be tented to prevent oxygen from collecting under the drape.

Source: AORN. (2013). Recommended practices for laser safety, pp. 146, 149-151; Recommended practices for safe environment of care, pp. 221-222. In *Perioperative Standards and Recommended Practices*. Denver: AORN, Inc.

Module 5: Malignant hyperthermia — Pages 217-219

Activity — Do You Know?

Circle the agents known to trigger malignant hyperthermia:

Desflurane   Enflurane   Halothane   Isoflurane   Sevoflurane   Succinylcholine

Source: Phillips, N. (2013). *Berry and Kohn's Operating Room Technique* (12 ed., p. 636). St. Louis: Mosby.

Activity — Critical Thinking

Which of the following is an early sign of malignant hyperthermia?

Tachycardia

Source: Phillips, N. (2013). *Berry and Kohn's Operating Room Technique* (12 ed., p. 636). St. Louis: Mosby.

Activity — Patient Scenario

Mr. J., a 70-year-old male comes to your hospital for a right total knee replacement. His past medical history includes a left inguinal hernia repair 20 years ago. He experienced no difficulties with anesthesia at that time. Significant history includes mild chronic obstructive lung disease and hypertension. He has smoked a pipe for the past 40 years and enjoys 1-2 mixed drinks several times a week. He is retired and considers himself in general good health. He has no known allergies. His current medications include lisinopril 12/25 once a day, a multi-vitamin, a maintenance inhaler, a nasal spray for his allergies, and one aspirin a day. The anesthesia care provider states his ASA score is 2. A rapid sequence induction is planned, because the patient had water with his medications this morning.

Mr. J. is transported to the OR suite at 0930. He is anesthetized, positioned, prepped, and draped. The surgical checklist is completed, including the time-out, with no issues identified. The surgery begins without incident.

At the same time that the knee prosthesis package is opened and the bone cement delivered to the field and mixed (1100), Mr. J.'s heart rate climbs to 120. The anesthesia care provider notes the patient is requiring more oxygen to maintain a normal oxygen saturation level. The circulating nurse notes that Mr. J.'s skin is becoming mottled with purple splotches. When the anesthesia care provider checks the placement of the endotracheal tube, she notes the jaw muscles are very tight. Mr. J.'s temperature is normal at 36.5°C.

1. Highlight the signs in the scenario indicative of MH.

- ***He is undergoing general anesthesia.***
- ***Mr. J.'s heart rate climbs to 120.***
- ***The anesthesia care provider notes the patient is requiring more oxygen to maintain a normal oxygen saturation level.***
- ***The circulating nurse notes that Mr. J.'s skin is becoming mottled with purple splotches.***
- ***When the anesthesia care provider checks the placement of the endotracheal tube, she notes the jaw muscles are very tight.***

Source: Phillips, N. (2013). *Berry and Kohn's Operating Room Technique* (12 ed., p. 636). St. Louis: Mosby.

2. What other conditions might you suspect?

- ***Allergic response to bone cement (methyl methacrylate).***
- ***Pulmonary embolism.***
- ***Allergic response to drug/anesthetic used intraoperatively.***

Module 6: Trauma — Pages 219-222

Activity — Critical Thinking

You work in a rural community hospital that provides care to the surrounding ranching community. The hospital has 22 beds, one OR, and a labor deck. Cesarean sections are performed in the main OR. The majority of your surgical population is adults. Two surgeons who are on staff perform general, orthopedic, and gynecologic surgeries. A neurosurgeon, Dr. H., comes in once a month from a major teaching facility and performs lumbar discectomies. An ENT surgeon from the neighboring county's hospital has a weekly schedule of tonsillectomies and myringotomies, which are performed on an outpatient basis. A certified registered nurse anesthetist (CRNA) is the primary anesthesia care provider.

You have completed your schedule for the day, including two lumbar discectomies with Dr. H., when the emergency department (ED) pages you stat. It is 1930 on a Friday evening. When you and Dr. H. arrive, you find the staff busy caring for the victims of a multi-car accident involving three people. The driver of one car managed to walk to a farmhouse to call for help. His injuries include a broken left clavicle and a contusion over his left eye. The driver of the other car is alert and oriented.

Her vital signs are:
>Pulse: 120 bpm
>Respirations: 20/min
>Blood pressure: 96/50 mmHg
>Pulse oximeter: 92% on 2L/O2
>Temperature: 36.5° C

She is guarding her right abdomen, which is rigid. She has an IV of 0.9% normal saline infusing through a 16 ga intravenous catheter in her right antecubital. A CBC has been sent to the lab. The ED doctor suspects intra-abdominal bleeding.

This patient's primary concern, however, is for her 9-year-old son. He was sleeping in the back seat, not wearing a seat belt, and was ejected from the vehicle. When emergency medical technicians arrived, the child was unresponsive with shallow respirations of 10/minute. He was intubated at the scene. Fluids are being administered through a left tibial intraosseous infusion. Moistened 4X4 sponges have been placed over an open head wound. The child responds with decerebrate posturing to painful stimuli. When Dr. H. removes the sponges, meninges are visible.

The child's vital signs are:
>Pulse: 120 bpm
>Respirations: Ventilated via bag-valve mask at 18 breaths/minute
>Blood pressure: Palpated at 48 mm Hg
>Pulse oximeter: 90%
>Temperature: 34.8° C
>Glasgow coma scale: 5

Based on your available resources, discuss your plan of care for these patients.

Responses will vary, but should address principles of triage and use of available resources:

This is a difficult situation and there is no one right answer. Resources and patient needs will need to be carefully evaluated.
- ***Two of the three accident victims need immediate surgical interventions. This facility has one operating room.***
- ***The nursing staff's experience is primarily with adults and well children.***

- *An experienced neurosurgeon is available in-house. A general surgeon is available.*
- *An anesthesia care provider is available in-house.*
- *OR staff is available in-house.*

Due to the extensive injuries sustained by the child and the resources available, the health care team may wish to consider transporting him to a level one trauma center and using the hospital OR team to perform an emergency laparotomy for the mother. In any case, additional resources are needed. The hospital's emergency disaster plan should be implemented to procure additional staff.

Source: Rothrock, J.C. (Ed.). (2011). *Alexander's Care of the Patient in Surgery* (14th ed., p. 1142). St. Louis: Mosby.

Activity — Word Scramble

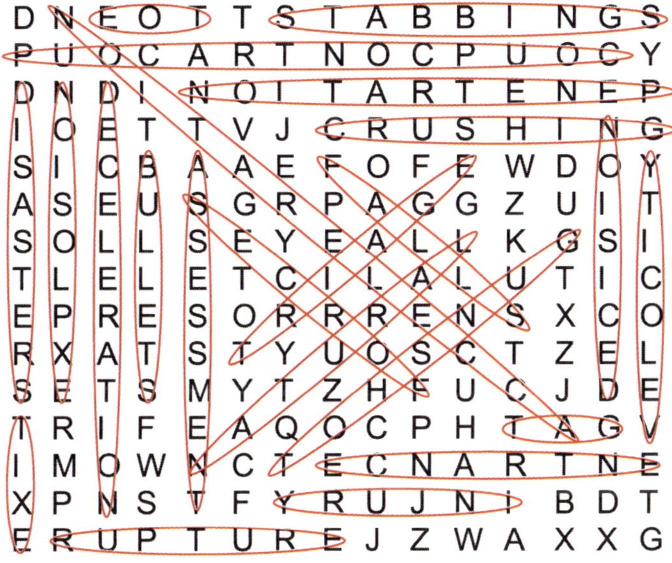

Module 7: Disasters — Pages 222-223

Activity — Matching

Match the bioterrorism agent to its modes of transmission. Answers may be used more than once.

Anthrax: *A, C, E*
Smallpox: *A, B, C, E*
Plague: *C, D, E*
Tularemia: *E, F, G, H*
Botulism: *E, G*

A. direct contact
B. indirect contact
C. droplet
D. flea or rodent bite

E. aerosol
F. infected animal tissue
G. contaminated food or water
H. arthropod bite

Source: Rothrock, J.C. (Ed.). (2011). *Alexander's Care of the Patient in Surgery* (14th ed., pp. 65-66). St. Louis: Mosby.

NOTES

CHAPTER 8:
Management of Personnel, Services, and Materials

> **Test Specifications:**
> *6% of CNOR test questions are based on Management of Personnel, Services, and Materials.*

Introduction

Patient care requires a complex interaction between the perioperative health care team and often highly technologically challenging equipment. It is the perioperative registered nurse's responsibility to ensure that all equipment, supplies, and the necessary expertise to safely care for the patient are assembled in the OR before the procedure begins. The Joint Commission (TJC) (2010) addresses the importance of having all immediate members of the health care team available prior to the beginning of the case as one way to avoid wrong site, wrong procedure, or wrong person surgery. Being prepared not only meets a TJC standard; it demonstrates fiscal responsibility and respect for both the patient's and the health care team's time, and influences patient safety issues such as infection control, pressure ulcers, and anesthetic risks.

This chapter reviews the perioperative nurse's role in the management of personnel, services, and materials and focuses on the following areas:

- The nurse's responsibilities in anticipating, obtaining, and managing the resources needed in operative and invasive procedures.
- Regulatory standards and voluntary guidelines that influence the scope of practice for the interdisciplinary team.
- Factors influencing product evaluation and cost containment.
- The role of health industry representatives and visitors in the perioperative setting.

Module 1: Management of the Interdisciplinary Team

All registered nurses, regardless of specialty, practice under the regulations outlined by their state boards of nursing. Every nurse must understand these regulations, as well as those from other governmental and regulatory agencies whose standards, policies, guidelines, and recommendations influence safe patient care.

An effective perioperative RN is also an effective manager. The special needs of the patient influence the degree of complexity of the procedure, the number of staff members present, supplies and equipment needed, skill sets required of other members of the health care team, and surgeon practice and preference. Organization, communication, and critical-thinking skills will expedite the safe and timely completion of the procedure and help to ensure optimal patient outcomes. Opportunities for mentoring are practically limitless as the perioperative nurse guides the team in providing safe patient care.

Competency Outcomes

To successfully complete the activities in this module, you will need to be able to:

1. Recognize the responsibility of the perioperative nurse in managing the perioperative environment.
2. Select appropriate tasks to delegate to members of the health care team.
3. Identify the regulations and standards affecting the nurse's practice in the perioperative setting.
4. Demonstrate a commitment to educating/mentoring health care team members.

Recommended Readings

AORN. (Dec. 2009). Position Statement: Responsibility for mentoring. Retrieved March 12, 2013, from http://www.aorn.org/Clinical_Practice/Position_Statements/Position_Statements.aspx.

Perioperative Standards and Recommended Practices. (2013):
- Exhibit B: Perioperative explications for the ANA Code of Ethics for Nurses, pp. 21-42.
- Guidance statement: Perioperative staffing.
- Guidance statement: Safe on-call practices in perioperative practice settings.

Alexander's Care of the Patient in Surgery. (2011, 14th ed.), Chapter 1: Concepts basic to perioperative nursing.

Berry and Kohn's Operating Room Technique. (2013, 12th ed.), Chapter 1: Perioperative education; Chapter 2: Foundations of perioperative patient care standards; Chapter 4: The perioperative patient care team and credentialing; Chapter 6: Administration of perioperative patient care services.

Competency for Safe Patient Care During Operative and Invasive Procedures. (2009), Chapter 4: Legal, regulatory, and ethical considerations.

National Council of State Boards of Nursing. (2013). *Delegation.* Retrieved March 12, 2013, from https://www.ncsbn.org/1625.htm

Key Words

Allied health care providers, competency, delegation, education, management, patient acuity, scope of practice, support personnel, unlicensed assistive personnel (UAP)

Activity — Do You Know?

1. Circle the following items that cannot be delegated.

Accountability	Task involving independent nursing judgment
Supervision	Making a nursing diagnosis
Responsibility	Providing extensive patient education
Routine task with a predictable outcome	Planning for patient discharge

2. Mark with an "X" all tasks that, according to the National Council of State Boards of Nursing, may be delegated by a perioperative registered nurse.

A.   Initial patient assessment to a licensed practical nurse (LPN). ____
B.   Standing order for a nursing assistant to insert an indwelling urinary catheter for all patients scheduled for a Cesarean section. ____
C.   Changing the rate of oxygen flow for a patient by the transporter.____
D.   Application of a tourniquet by a newly hired RNFA whose competency in this task is unknown.____
E.   Interpretation of an EKG by the ward clerk on a telemetry unit.____

Activity — Critical Thinking

It is 11:30 on a Friday night. Mr. K., 57 years old, has been admitted to the emergency department of a small community hospital. He has been in a motorcycle accident. His medication history includes warfarin (Coumadin) for atrial fibrillation. He had a large dinner at 7:00 PM.

Diagnostic exams include a computed tomography (CT) scan and x-rays. The CT scan shows bleeding from the spleen. He is cold, clammy, and very pale. His vital signs currently are:

BP: 84/40 mmHg
Respirations: 22 per minute
Pulse: 120 bpm
Temperature: 97.8° F tympanic membrane
Pulse oximeter: 93% on 2 L O_2 per nasal cannula
Pain: 10 on a scale of 0 to 10

His blood pressure is being maintained by rapid infusion of intravenous crystalloids and whole blood while the trauma surgeon and OR team are called in. The OR call team consists of an anesthesia care provider, one RN, and one surgical technologist. The post-anesthesia care unit nurse is typically called in when the surgeon begins closing.

BL is the only perioperative nurse on duty.

1. What options could BL consider in arranging for additional personnel to assist with Mr. K.'s care?

2. What other blood products might BL expect to need for this case?

3. What additional supplies or equipment might be anticipated to be needed in the OR to be prepared for this case?

4. What outside services/resources should be requested?

"Go To" Activity — Skill Building

Look up your state board's rules and regulations governing nursing practice.
  (National Council of State Boards of Nursing [2013]. Boards of Nursing. Retrieved March 12, 2013, from https://www.ncsbn.org/boards.htm)

What is your facility's policy on overtime/scheduled call? Compare it to AORN's guidance statement on safe on-call practices.

Review and update if necessary your facility's policy on emergency procedures.

Additional Readings/ Resources

Hemingway, M., Freehan, M., & Morrissey, L. (2010). Expanding the role of nonclinical personnel in the OR. *AORN Journal, 91*(6), 753-761.

National Council of State Boards of Nursing. (2011, Jan.). NCSBN Model Practice Act and Model Nursing Administrative Rules. Retrieved March 12, 2013, from https://www.ncsbn.org/Model_Nursing_Practice_Act_March2011.pdf

Case Study Activity

A sample preference card with basic instrumentation/supplies for a laparoscopic cholecystectomy is shown below. Based on Mrs. M.'s special needs, what additional resources/equipment will be needed?

PROCEDURE: LAPAROSCOPY CHOLECYSTECTOMY
TEXT: NOTES

POSITION: SUPINE
* * * CHECK BEFORE YOU OPEN TROCARS * * *
HAVE X-RAY GOWNS AVAILABLE
HAVE 5.5MM X 7.5 MM TROCARS AVAILABLE FOR EACH CASE
* * * * *
VIDEO TOWERS X2 AT TOP OF BED - ELECTROSURGICAL UNIT AT FOOT - HAVE BED YOU CAN X-RAY THROUGH
LOCAL: AT BEGINNING OF CASE
* * * * *
WARM IRRIGATION PLEASE
WARMS LENS PRIOR TO CASE
SEQUENTIAL COMPRESSION STOCKINGS, UPPER BODY WARMER
* * * * *
USES ONE 10/12MM TROCAR, THREE 5MM, 7.5MM LENGTH
5MM 0 DEGREE LENS
* * * * *
LIKES "S" RETRACTORS, LIKES MARYLAND DISSECTOR AND HOOK CAUTERY

Item Name	**Item Name**
BLANKET WARMING UPPER	ELECTROSURGICAL UNIT
PAD ARMBOARD OR 20X8X2	VIDEO TOWER
PREP SKIN CHLORHEXIDINE 26ML	WARM AIR BLANKET
	C-ARM
PACK GENERAL LAPAROSCOPIC	SEQUENTIAL COMPRESSION STOCKINGS
DRAPE C ARM SHOWER CAP	HARMONIC SCALPEL
TOWELS, DISPOSABLE	
GOWN SURGICAL STD XL	**SUTURE**
GLOVE SURG POWDER FREE	VICRYL 3-0 27IN SH J416H
MARKER SKIN REG TIP	VICRYL 0 27 IN CT2 J27OH
STOPCOCK 5-WAY LG BODY	MONCRYL 4-0 PS2 Y426H
PEANUT ENDO	VICRYL 0 27IN UR6 J603H
SYRINGE 20ML	
TIP SUC IRR SMOKEVAC	
TUBING INSUF ENDO	
KIT CLOSURE	
APPLCLIP ENDO	

INSTRUMENTS	**Medications**		**Dose**
LAP CHOLE INSTRUMENTS		SOD CHL 0.9% FOR IRRIGATION	3000
LAP CHOLE SOFT TISSUE SET		SOD CHL 0.9% FOR IRRIGATION	1000
LAPAROSCOPIC LENS, 5MM & CORD		SOD CHL 0.9% IV	1000
INSUFFLATOR CORD		BUPIVACAINE / EPINEPHRINE 0.25%	50
		RENOGRAFIN 60	50
		TISSUE SEALANT	1

Text: GENERAL SUPPLIES
ALWAYS CHOLANGIOGRAM
ALWAYS OPEN 5MM TROCARS X 3, 10MM TROCAR X 1

Module 2: Principles of Product Evaluation and Cost Containment

The health care facility relies heavily on its nurses' judicious use of supplies and equipment to remain fiscally solvent. Although the OR is considered a revenue generating department, it is also one of the most expensive in terms of capital and supply needs.

The OR plays a large role in contributing to the estimated 4 billion pounds of waste generated by health care facilities annually (AORN, 2013, p. 1). Minimizing waste saves money and allows for more resources to be available for more patients.

The combination of cost-containment and environmental factors encourages the re-use of supplies whenever safely possible. As end-users, the perioperative RN is in a unique position to recommend the purchase and use of equipment and supplies that are safe, cost-effective, and environmentally friendly.

Competency Outcomes

To successfully complete the activities in this module, you will need to be able to:

1. Identify criteria used in selecting products.
2. Analyze the financial impact of the product on the facility.
3. Assess the effect of proposed product purchases on the environment.

Recommended Readings

Perioperative Standards and Recommended Practices. (2013):
- Recommended practices: Sterilization.
- Recommended practices: Product selection.

Berry and Kohn's Operating Room Technique. (2013, 12th ed.), pp. 97, 213, 300-301, 487-488.

Key Words

Cost containment, environmental consciousness (go green), fiscal responsibility, product evaluation, product selection, recycling, resource conservation, single-use device (SUD), supply management

---

"Go To" Activity — Check It Out!

Go to Question # 21, Reprocessing single-use items, under the Perioperative question of the week tab on your CD for a critical-thinking question related to reprocessing opened but unused sterile items.

Activity — Critical Thinking

Your facility is considering purchasing a new electrosurgical dispersive unit.

1. Who should be on the product evaluation committee?

2. What should be included in the selection criteria for this device?

3. What factors are to be considered in determining the impact of this product on the environment?

Additional Readings/Resources

Burlingame, B. (2009). Decreasing the effect of perioperative care on the environment; Starting an OR recycling program. *AORN Journal, 90*(3), 443-446.

Conrardy, J., Hillanbrand, M., Myers, S., & Nussbaum, G.F. (2010). Reducing medical waste. *AORN Journal, 91*(6), 711-721.

Mejia, E., & Sattler, B. (2009). Starting a health care system green team. *AORN Journal, 90*(1), 33-40.

Ogden, J. (2009). Blue wrap recycling: It can be done! *AORN Journal, 89*(4), 739-743.

Pennington, C., & DeRienzo, N.R. (2010). An effective process for making decisions about major operating room purchases. *AORN Journal, 91*(3), 341-349.

"Go To" Activity — Skill Building

Spend an hour with the material management person from your facility. Review the costs for commonly used equipment and supplies (e.g., instruments, suture, OR furniture). Discuss the process of purchasing supplies and capital equipment.

Volunteer to sit on your facility's product selection committee as a representative from the perioperative department.

Module 3: Management of Ancillary Personnel in the Perioperative Setting

People who are not typically considered members of the health care team may nevertheless be included in the operative or invasive procedure. As equipment and procedures become more complex, industry specialists frequently assist the perioperative team with products as they are being used. Students from a variety of specialties benefit from exposure to surgery as part of their learning experience. Patient safety, privacy, and confidentiality need to be maintained regardless of the makeup of the health care team.

Competency Outcomes

To successfully complete the activities in this module, you will need to be able to:

1. Manage health care industry representative presence in the procedural setting.
2. Assess appropriateness of visitors in the perioperative area based on patient safety and privacy issues.

Recommended Readings

Perioperative Standards and Recommended Practices. (2013).
- Guidance statement: Role of the health care industry representative.
- Recommended practices: Sterilization.

Alexander's Care of the Patient in Surgery. (2011, 14th ed.), Chapter 1: Concepts basic to perioperative nursing; Chapter 2: Patient safety and risk management.

AORN Position Statement: Allied health care providers and support personnel in the perioperative practice setting. (Feb. 2011). Retrieved March 13, 2013, from http://www.aorn.org/Clinical_Practice/Position_Statements/Position_Statements.aspx.

AORN Position Statement: Value of clinical learning activities in the perioperative setting in undergraduate nursing curricula. (Dec. 2009). Retrieved March 13, 2013, from http://www.aorn.org/Clinical_Practice/Position_Statements/Position_Statements.aspx.

Berry and Kohn's Operating Room Technique. (2013, 12th ed.), pp. 2-5, 17-18, 42, 51-55, 325-326.

Key Words

Accountability, ethics, health care industry representative, loaner instrumentation, patient rights, patient privacy, vendor, visitor

Activity — What Do You Do?

A vendor arrives at your OR at 0715 with a new hip implant system that your hospital does not carry. He states the surgeon "just wants to try it." He asks to scrub in so that he may better assist the surgeon in placing the implant.

1. What are the issues identified?

2. How would you respond?

"Go To" Activity — Check It Out!

Go to Question # 39, Student placement in the OR, under the Perioperative question of the week tab on your CD for a critical-thinking exercise.

"Go To" Activity — Skill Building

Review your facility policy on visitors in OR and compare it to AORN's Recommended Practices on Safe Environment of Care, Recommendations I and II.

Visit your medical staffing office to learn about privileging process for vendors.

Review your facility's consent form for patient rights related to notification of visitor presence in the OR and right of refusal.

Ask your unit educator to share the syllabus and expected outcomes for student experiences.

Case Study Activity

A student has been assigned to your room to observe Mrs. M.'s surgery. What are your responsibilities as:

• an advocate for Mrs. M.?

• a preceptor for the student?

Additional Readings/Resources:

Cooper, K., & Bowers, B. (2006). Demystifying the OR for baccalaureate nursing students. *AORN Journal, 84*(5), 827-836.

Girard, N. J. (2006). Like it or not, you are a role model. *AORN Journal, 84*(1), 13-15.

Huter-Kunish, G. (2009). Processing loaner instruments in an ambulatory surgery center. *AORN Journal, 89*(5), 861-866. Bonus: Exam questions follow the article.

Pape, T. M. (2007). Creating an inviting perioperative learning experience. *AORN Journal, 85*(2), 354-366.

Rickets, D.L., & Gray, S. E. (2010). Improving associate degree nursing students' perioperative clinical observation experiences. *AORN Journal, 91*(3), 383-389.

Seavey, R. (2010). Reducing the risks associated with loaner instrumentation and implants. *AORN Journal, 92*(3), 322-331.

Sigsby, L.M., Selzer, J., & Wilson, T.K. (2006). A successful nursing student practicum in an ambulatory surgery center. *AORN Journal, 84*(2), 219-232.

Chapter Summary

Effective management of personnel, services, and materials is the cornerstone of assuring the patient a safe and efficient perioperative experience. Following established institutional policies and procedures, professional standards, recommended practices, and guidelines will assist in procuring the resources needed to provide safe care for every patient.

Glossary

Accountability — Being responsible and answerable for actions or inactions of self or others in the context of delegation. Accountability cannot be delegated.

Code of ethics — Guidelines regarding professional behavior and ethical decision-making. AORN has developed "explications for perioperative nursing" for each statement in the ANA code to provide the context within which perioperative nurses can make ethical decisions.

Competency — Possessing the knowledge and skills necessary to safely perform a task.

Delegation — Transferring to a competent individual the authority to perform a selected nursing task in a selected situation. The nurse retains accountability for the delegation. Delegation is limited to situations in which the patient is stable and where the outcome of the delegated task is predictable. It is the responsibility of the delegator to verify competency of the delegatee. Delegation of care is only allowed within the RN scope of practice.

Delegator — The person making the delegation.

Delegatee (also called delegate) — The person receiving the delegation.

Health care industry representative — Health care industry employees who provide services in the perioperative setting including clinical consultants, sales representatives, technicians, and repair/maintenance personnel.

Patient rights — Every patient has the right to seek and receive health care provided with respect for his or her self-image and privacy, regardless of race, religion, or culture.

Supervision — The provision of guidance or direction, evaluation and follow-up by the licensed nurse for accomplishment of a nursing task delegated to unlicensed assistive personnel. Supervision cannot be delegated.

Unlicensed assistive personnel (UAP) — Any unlicensed person, regardless of title, to whom nursing tasks are delegated.

References

American Nurses Association (ANA). (2001). Code of ethics for nurses with interpretive statements. Retrieved March 13, 2013, from http://nursingworld.org/MainMenuCategories/EthicsStandards/CodeofEthicsforNurses/Code-of-Ethics.pdf.

AORN. (2013). Exhibit B: Perioperative explications for the ANA Code of Ethics for nurses. In *Perioperative Standards and Recommended Practices*. Denver: AORN, Inc.

AORN. (2013). AORN Guidance statement on role of the health care industry representative. In *Perioperative Standards and Recommended Practices*. Denver: AORN, Inc.

AORN. (2013). AORN Recommended practices for product selection. In *Perioperative Standards and Recommended Practices*. Denver: AORN, Inc.

AORN. (2011). Position Statement: Creating a practice environment of safety. Retrieved March 12, 2013, from http://www.aorn.org/Clinical_Practice/Position_Statements/Position_Statements.aspx.

AORN. (2011). Position Statement: Environmental responsibility. Retrieved April 23, 2013, from http://www.aorn.org/Clinical_Practice/Position_Statements/Position_Statements.aspx.

The Joint Commission. (2012). Introduction to the Universal Protocol for Preventing Wrong Site, Wrong Procedure, and Wrong Person Surgery™. In *The Joint Commission Comprehensive Accreditation and Certification Manual E-dition*. Retrieved Feb. 21, 2013, from http://www.jointcommission.org/assets/1/18/TJC_Annual_Report_2012.pdf.

National Council of State Boards of Nursing. (2013). *Delegation*. Retrieved March 13, 2013, from https://www.ncsbn.org/1625.htm.

Phillips, N. (2013). *Berry and Kohn's Operating Room Technique* (12th ed.). St. Louis: Mosby.

Phippen, M. L., Ulmer, B.C., & Wells, M.P. (2009). *Competency for Safe Patient Care During Operative and Invasive Procedures*. Denver:CCI.

Rothrock, J.C. (Ed.). (2011). *Alexander's Care of the Patient in Surgery* (14th ed.). St. Louis: Mosby.

Answers to Chapter 8 Activities

Module I: Management of the interdisciplinary team — Pages 235-239

Activity — Do You Know?

1. Circle the following items that cannot be delegated.

Accountability	*Task involving independent nursing judgment*
Supervision	*Making a nursing diagnosis*
Providing extensive patient education	*Planning for patient discharge*

Sources: AORN. (2013). *Perioperative Standards and Recommended Practices*, Exhibit B: Perioperative explications for the ANA Code of Ethics for Nurses, p. 33; Rothrock, J.C. (Ed.). (2011). *Alexander's Care of the Patient in Surgery* (14th ed.). St. Louis: Mosby, p. 10.

2. Mark with an "X" all tasks that, according to the National Council of State Boards of Nursing, may be delegated by a perioperative registered nurse.

A. Initial patient assessment to a licensed practical nurse (LPN)
B. Standing order for a nursing assistant to insert an indwelling urinary catheter in all patients scheduled for a Cesarean section
C. Changing the rate of oxygen flow for a patient by the transporter
D. Application of a tourniquet by a newly hired RNFA whose competency in this task is unknown
E. Interpretation of an EKG by the ward clerk on a telemetry unit
Answer: None of the above.

Source: National Council of State Boards of Nursing. (2013). *Delegation*. Retrieved March 13, 2013, from https://www.ncsbn.org/1625.htm.

Activity — Critical Thinking

It is 11:30 on a Friday night. Mr. K., 57 years old, has been admitted to the emergency department of a small community hospital. He has been in a motorcycle accident. His medication history includes warfarin (Coumadin) for atrial fibrillation. He had a large dinner at 7:00 PM.

Diagnostic exams include a computed tomography (CT) scan and x-rays. The CT scan shows bleeding from the spleen. He is cold, clammy, and very pale. His vital signs currently are:

    BP: 84/40 mmHg
    Respirations: 22 per minute
    Pulse: 120 bpm
    Temperature: 97.8° F tympanic membrane
    Pulse oximeter: 93% on 2 L O_2 per nasal cannula
    Pain: 10 on a scale of 0 to 10

His blood pressure is being maintained by rapid infusion of intravenous crystalloids and whole blood while the trauma surgeon and OR team are called in. The OR call team consists of an anesthesia care provider, one RN, and one surgical technologist. The postanesthesia care unit nurse is typically called in when the surgeon begins closing.

BL is the only perioperative nurse on duty.

1. What options could BL consider in arranging for additional personnel to assist with Mr. K.'s care?

Responses to Consider:

Because Mr. K. is hemorrhaging severely from his spleen, adequate fluid resuscitation and blood product administration is essential for a positive outcome. BL identifies that he will need additional resources to effectively manage Mr. K. in the OR. Options include:

- ***If there is no backup perioperative OR nurse on call, ask the postanesthesia care unit (PACU) RN on call to come in early.***
- ***Call the nursing supervisor/house manager for assistance.***
- ***If the ED is not too busy, an RN could assist with fluid resuscitation and administration of blood products.***
- ***Call the OR manager.***
- ***Ask the nursing supervisor/house manager to call other OR staff RNs to come in.***

BL has an opportunity to improve the on-call system for this OR for future emergency cases. By discussing the situation with the surgical services administrator or OR manager and/or offering to lead a team to identify potential solutions and make a recommendation to the administration, a plan can be developed to handle similar situations.

2. What other blood products might BL expect to need for this case?

In addition to fluid volume replacement with IV fluids, the nurse can expect Mr. K. to receive additional plasma expanders and packed cells.

3. What additional supplies or equipment might be anticipated to be needed in the OR to be prepared for this case?

- ***Suction should be set up and readily available because of Mr. K.'s full stomach and the possibility of vomiting and risk for aspiration. BL should have a nasogastric tube available for insertion. BL should be prepared to assist with a rapid-sequence induction, including cricoid pressure.***

- ***Due to severe hemorrhaging from the spleen and the patient's history of anticoagulant use, the following additional supplies and equipment should be available: additional IV fluids, volume expanders, a blood pump, a fluid warmer, blood filters, vascular clamps and suture, an autologous blood transfusion device, a rapid infuser, an arterial line set-up, and extra laparotomy pads and x-ray detectable 4X4 sponges.***

4. What outside services/resources should be requested?

A staff member from the blood bank or the house manager may be able to bring extra units of blood, or bring several units in a cooler. A lab technician could be available to draw blood for arterial blood gases, hemoglobin and hematocrit, and clotting factors. Additional personnel are needed to operate the autologous blood transfusion device and rapid infuser. The trauma surgeon needs an assistant, such as a registered nurse first assistant (RNFA), a physician's assistant (PA), or another physician.

Case Study Activity

A sample preference card with basic instrumentation/supplies for a laparoscopic cholecystectomy is shown on the next page. Based on Mrs. M.'s special needs, what additional resources/equipment will be needed?

List is not all-inclusive:

Portable x-ray	***Extra help for positioning/transfer***
C-arm	***Send for patient bed***
Sleds/arm positioners	***Notify radiology***
Extra-long veress needle	***Extra-large blood pressure cuff***
Laparotomy set for possible open procedure	***Glucometer***

PROCEDURE: LAPAROSCOPY CHOLECYSTECTOMY

TEXT: NOTES

POSITION: SUPINE
* * * CHECK BEFORE YOU OPEN TROCARS * * *
HAVE X-RAY GOWNS AVAILABLE
HAVE 5.5MM X 7.5 MM TROCARS AVAILABLE FOR EACH CASE
* * * * *
VIDEO TOWERS X2 AT TOP OF BED - ELECTROSURGICAL UNIT AT FOOT - HAVE BED YOU CAN X-RAY THROUGH
LOCAL: AT BEGINNING OF CASE
* * * * *
WARM IRRIGATION PLEASE
WARMS LENS PRIOR TO CASE
SEQUENTIAL COMPRESSION STOCKINGS, UPPER BODY WARMER
* * * * *
USES ONE 10/12MM TROCAR, THREE 5MM, 7.5MM LENGTH
5MM 0 DEGREE LENS
* * * * *
LIKES "S" RETRACTORS, LIKES MARYLAND DISSECTOR AND HOOK CAUTERY

Item Name	**Item Name**	
BLANKET WARMING UPPER	ELECTROSURGICAL UNIT	
PAD ARMBOARD OR 20X8X2	VIDEO TOWER	
PREP SKIN CHLORHEXIDINE 26ML	WARM AIR BLANKET	
	C-ARM	
PACK GENERAL LAPAROSCOPIC	SEQUENTIAL COMPRESSION STOCKINGS	
DRAPE C ARM SHOWER CAP	HARMONIC SCALPEL	
TOWELS, DISPOSABLE		
GOWN SURGICAL STD XL	**SUTURE**	
GLOVE SURG POWDER FREE	VICRYL 3-0 27IN SH J416H	
MARKER SKIN REG TIP	VICRYL 0 27 IN CT2 J27OH	
STOPCOCK 5-WAY LG BODY	MONCRYL 4-0 PS2 Y426H	
PEANUT ENDO	VICRYL 0 27IN UR6 J603H	
SYRINGE 20ML		
TIP SUC IRR SMOKEVAC		
TUBING INSUF ENDO		
KIT CLOSURE		
APPLCLIP ENDO		

INSTRUMENTS	**Medications**	**Dose**
LAP CHOLE INSTRUMENTS	SOD CHL 0.9% FOR IRRIGATION	3000
LAP CHOLE SOFT TISSUE SET	SOD CHL 0.9% FOR IRRIGATION	1000
LAPAROSCOPIC LENS, 5MM & CORD	SOD CHL 0.9% IV	1000
INSUFFLATOR CORD	BUPIVACAINE / EPINEPHRINE 0.25%	50
	RENOGRAFIN 60	50
	TISSUE SEALANT	1

Text: GENERAL SUPPLIES

ALWAYS CHOLANGIOGRAM
ALWAYS OPEN 5MM TROCARS X 3, 10MM TROCAR X 1

Module 2: Principles of product evaluation and cost containment — Pages 240-241

Activity — Critical Thinking

Your facility is considering purchasing a new electrosurgical dispersive unit.

1. Who should be on the product evaluation committee?

Anyone using the device, educating others on the safe use of the device, or involved with supply procurement/purchasing, including:

- *Staff RNs*
- *Material manager*
- *Financial director*
- *Surgical services administration*
- *Staff development educator*

2. What should be included in the selection criteria?

- *Patient safety*
- *Cost*
- *Compatibility with electrosurgical unit*
- *Warranties/contractual agreements*
- *Procedure-related requirements*
- *Latex free*
- *Ease of use*

3. What factors are to be considered in determining the impact of this product on the environment?

- *Are the product and packaging made of recycled materials?*
- *Can the product be recycled?*
- *What method is used for disposal?*
- *Are packaging and shipping materials kept to a minimum?*

Source: AORN. (2013). Recommended Practices: Product selection, pp. 197-201. In *Perioperative Standards and Recommended Practices*. Denver: AORN.

Module 3: Management of ancillary personnel in the perioperative setting — Pages 242-244

Activity — What Do You Do?

A vendor arrives at your OR at 0715 with a new hip implant system that your hospital does not carry. He states the surgeon "just wants to try it." He asks to scrub in so that he may better assist the surgeon in placing the implant.

1. What are the issues identified? *(possible answers)*

- *Patient consent for procedure*
- *Education of team on new system*
- *Credentials/privileges for vendor*
- *Sterilization of implants delivered day of surgery*

2. How would you respond? *(possible answers)*

- *The surgeon must discuss plan for new instrumentation and get consent from patient.*
- *Loaner instrumentation must be processed in accordance with safe sterilization practices; this may necessitate rescheduling case for a later time.*
- *Medical staffing office must be contacted and credentials verified for industry representative.*
- *Staff must be educated on new system.*

Source: AORN. (2013). Guidance statement: The role of the health care industry representative, pp. 541-542; Recommended practices for cleaning and care of surgical instruments and powered equipment, Recommendation III, p. 486. In *Perioperative Standards and Recommended Practices*. Denver: AORN.

Case Study Activity

A student has been assigned to your room to observe Mrs. M.'s surgery. What are your responsibilities as:

(Answers are representative and are not meant to be all-inclusive.)

- an advocate for Mrs. M.?

  Ask Mrs. M. for her permission to allow the student to observe her surgery.
  Maintain confidentiality of patient documentation.
  Maintain patient privacy during transfer, positioning, and prepping.
  Share and discuss only pertinent information related to Mrs. M.'s care.
  Check with unit educator/manager to ensure student has met academic and facility requirements for placement at the facility.

- a preceptor for the student?

  Introduce student to other members of the health care team.
  Facilitate the work environment to make it conducive to learning.
  Model professional behavior.
  Check with unit educator/manager to ensure student has met academic and facility requirements for placement at the facility.
  Obtain objectives and goals for clinical experience and work with student to meet as many as possible.

Sources: AORN. (2013). *Perioperative Standards and Recommended Practices*, Exhibit B: Perioperative explications for the ANA Code of Ethics for Nurses, pp. 28, 36-38. A0RN. (Dec. 2009). Position statement: Responsibility for mentoring. Retrieved March 13, 2013, from http://www.aorn.org/Clinical_Practice/Position_Statements/Position_Statements.aspx.

NOTES

CHAPTER 9:
Professional Accountability

Introduction

Society holds nurses, individually and collectively, accountable for acting in the public's best interest. Professional accountability, however, goes beyond being an exemplary clinician; a profession is more than a job. A profession includes the expectation of commitment to personal excellence and professional involvement that rises above the expectations of the workplace.

This chapter will help you identify the components of professional responsibility and accountability, and the resources available for functioning effectively as a professional perioperative nurse.

Module 1: Principles of Social Policy

The nursing profession is defined both legally and by expert practice recommendations. Statutes, regulations, standards, and guidelines that govern the practice of professional nursing are developed by legal entities and experts in the field to protect and promote the welfare of the patients nurses serve. Appendix D provides a list of frequently referenced agencies.

"Scope of practice" relates to WHAT a nurse can do, and "standards of practice" describe HOW the nurse is expected to practice. Standards describe what experts consider to be the best way to approach clinical challenges to facilitate the best patient outcomes.

Competency Outcomes

To successfully complete the activities in this module, you will need to be able to:

1. Examine regulatory agencies' contributions to providing guidance in protecting the patient.
2. Review your state's nurse practice act.
3. Differentiate between scope of practice and standards of practice.

Recommended Reading

Alexander's Care of the Patient in Surgery. (2011, 14th ed.), Chapter 1: Concepts basic to perioperative nursing.

Perioperative Standards and Recommended Practices, (2013):
* Standards of perioperative nursing, pp. 3-17.
* Exhibit B: Perioperative explications for the ANA code of ethics for nurses, pp. 21-42.

> **"Go To" Activity — Check It Out!**
>
> Go to Question # 34, Scope of practice, under the Perioperative question of the week tab on your CD for a critical-thinking question.

Berry and Kohn's Operating Room Technique. (2013, 12th ed.), Chapter 2: Foundations of perioperative patient care standards; Chapter 6: Administration of perioperative patient services.

Competency for Safe Patient Care During Operative and Invasive Procedures. (2009), Chapter 1: Systems-in-contingency: A conceptual model; Chapter 4: Legal, regulatory, and ethical considerations.

Key Words

Administrative agency, best practice, board of nursing, community standard, delegation, evidence-based practice, guidelines, nurse practice act, position statement, recommended practices, regulation, scope of practice, standard, statute

> **"Go To" Activity — Skill Building**
>
> Obtain a copy of the Nurse Practice Act for your state. Compare its scope of practice with your current job description.

Additional Reading/Resources

AORN. (2010). State continuing education requirements. *AORN Journal, 92*(6), S120-S122.

Becker, C. (2006). A license without borders. *AORN Journal, 83*(4), 958.

Glover, D.E., Newkirk, L.E., Cole, L.M., Walker, T.J., et al. (2006). Perioperative clinical nurse specialist role delineation: A systematic review. *AORN Journal, 84*(6), 1017-1030.

Schroeder, J.L. (2008). Acute care nurse practitioner: An advanced practice role for RN First Assistants. *AORN Journal, 87*(6), 1205-1215.

Stannard, D. (2009). Nursing ethics and professional responsibility in advanced practice. *AORN Journal, 90*(2), 295-296.

Activity — Matching

Match the agency with the service it provides (below).

Association of periOperative Registered Nurses (AORN) _______

Centers for Disease Control and Prevention (CDC) _______

Centers for Medicare and Medicaid services (CMS) _______

Food and Drug Administration (FDA) _______

Health Information Portability and Accountability Act (HIPAA) _______

The Joint Commission (TJC) _______

State board of nursing _______

Surgical Care Improvement Project (SCIP) _______

Occupational Safety and Health Administration (OSHA) _______

A. Ensures a safe and healthy workplace that would not subject workers to hazards that could result in physical harm or death

B. Identifies preventable conditions and prevents hospitals for billing for these costs

C. Addresses confidentiality of patient information in the medical record and consent processes for access to patients' health information

D. Provides information on infectious diseases

E. Establishes National Safety Patient Goals and conducts surveys to monitor compliance

F. Combination of governmental/non-governmental organizations focused on improving care by reducing surgical complications

G. Regulates medical devices and pharmaceuticals

H. Professional organization that empowers perioperative nurses with education, networking opportunities, and standards for nursing practice

I. Protects the public's health and welfare by overseeing and ensuring the safe practice of nursing

Module 2: Resources for Professional Growth

Included in the defining characteristics of a professional is the responsibility to evaluate one's own nursing practice in relation to professional practice standards (e.g., AORN's standards and recommended practices) and relevant state and federal regulations. Competency is defined as the application of the "knowledge, skills, and interpersonal abilities in fulfilling functions to provide safe, individualized patient care" (Phillips, 2013, p. 1).

Competency is measured in many different ways, starting with state nursing boards, which validate minimal competency for all nurses to provide safe nursing care. Other methods of assessing competent performance include:

- Direct observation by one's peers or supervisor.
- Audits of patient health care records and other documents.
- Compliance with local, state, and federal regulations.
- Specialty certification.

Competency Outcomes

To successfully complete the activities in this module, you will need to be able to:

1. Define competency.
2. Incorporate best practice standards into professional practice.
3. Identify resources for professional growth.

Recommended Reading

Alexander's Care of the Patient in Surgery. (2011, 14th ed.), Chapter 1: Concepts basic to perioperative nursing.

Perioperative Standards and Recommended Practices. (2013):
- Standards of perioperative nursing, pp. 3-17.
- Exhibit B: Perioperative explications for the ANA code of ethics for nurses, pp. 21-42.

Berry and Kohn's Operating Room Technique. (2013, 12th ed.), Chapter 1: Perioperative education; Chapter 2: Foundations of perioperative patient care standards; Chapter 4: The perioperative patient care team and professional credentialing.

Competency for Safe Patient Care During Operative and Invasive Procedures. (2009), Chapter 2: Competency assessment; Chapter 4: The perioperative patient care team and professional credentialing.

Key Words

Assessment, best practice, competency, competent, continuing education, life long learning, professional organization

<table>
<tr><td>

"Go To" Activity — Scavenger Hunt: AORN Web Site

Locate the following resources on the AORN web site (www.aorn.org):
- Specialty assemblies
- OR Nurselink
- Tool kits
- AORN library
- Professional development
- Benefits of membership

</td><td>

"Go To" Activity — Scavenger Hunt: CCI Web Site

Locate the following resources on the CCI web site (www.cc-institute.org):

- *CNOR Candidate Handbook*
- CCI Study Plan
- Learn about the exam
- Webinars

</td></tr>
</table>

"Go To" Activity — Skill Building

Review the competency assessment tools used in your facility. How are annual competencies determined? How is successfully meeting the criteria in the competency measured?

Attend an AORN chapter meeting; if already a member, volunteer for a committee or board position.

Create a study group for other staff members who are preparing for the CNOR exam.

Additional Reading/Resources

AORN. (2010). *Perioperative competencies, position descriptions, and evaluation tools.* Denver: AORN.

AORN. (2009). Magnet™ hospitals: The power to attract and retain top OR nurses. *AORN Journal, 90*(4), 609.

Banschbach, S.K. (2008). Making the most of our association's opportunities. *AORN Journal, 87*(5), 895-898.

Byrne, M., Schroeter, K., & Mower, J. (2010). Perioperative specialty certification: The CNOR as evidence for Magnet™ excellence. *AORN Journal, 91*(5), 618-622.

Gillespie, B.M., & Hamlin, L. (2009). A synthesis of the literature on "competence" as it applies to perioperative nursing. *AORN Journal, 90*(2), 245-258.

Jurkovich, P., Karpiuk, K., & King, C.A. (2010). Magnet™ recognition: Examples of perioperative excellence. *AORN Journal, 91*(2), 292-299.

Stobinski, J.X. (2008). Perioperative nursing competency. *AORN Journal, 88*(3), 417-436.

Sullivan, D., & Stevenson, D. (2009). Promoting professional organization involvement. *AORN Journal, 90*(4), 575-579.

Module 3: Participation in Quality Improvement Activities

The quality improvement process is ingrained in health care systems today and is driven by many national initiatives through reportable quality indicators. Quality improvement projects are often based on best practice recommendations. In turn, the results of these projects can be incorporated into actions to support changes to practice. The success of any quality improvement process hinges on the participation and support of those directly involved in providing patient care, including the nurse who cares for the patient during surgery.

Competency Outcomes

To successfully complete the activities in this module, you will need to be able to:

1. Identify the role of the perioperative nurse in quality improvement.
2. Apply a change template to common perioperative problems.

Recommended Reading

Alexander's Care of the Patient in Surgery. (2011, 14th ed.), Chapter 1: Concepts basic to perioperative nursing.

Perioperative Standards and Recommended Practices. (2013):
* Standards of perioperative nursing, pp. 3-17.
* Exhibit B: Perioperative explications for the ANA code of ethics for nurses, pp. 21-42.

Berry and Kohn's Operating Room Technique. (2013, 12th ed.), Chapter 2: Foundations of perioperative patient care standards; Chapter 6: Administration of perioperative patient services.

Competency for Safe Patient Care During Operative and Invasive Procedures. (2009), Chapter 3: Performance improvement.

Key Words

Audit, best practice, change, evidence-based practice, information literacy, measures, performance improvement, plan-do-study-act, shared governance

Activity — Critical Thinking

Write the step in the appropriate section for the quality improvement project:

Plan	**Do**	**Study**	**Act**

___________ Data was collected for 3 months by staff in 0730 cases. An audit tool was completed. The top 5 reasons for a late start were analyzed.

___________ Data showed that most cases were late due to insufficient staff to handle volume of patients in pre-admissions testing for day-of laboratory work.

___________ Steps to address findings include:
- Possibility of increasing number of pre-admission staff for morning shift
- Assess workload to determine tasks that could be delegated to another person

___________ The objective of this project is to decrease the number of late start 0730 cases. Promoting efficient use of time will allow the following cases to also begin on time, increase patient and surgeon satisfaction, and decrease the amount of overtime for staff. Data will be collected related to late starts, type of case, surgeon, and cause of late start.

Additional Reading/Resources

Hanson, D., Hoss, B.L., & Wesorick, B. (2008). Evaluating the evidence: Guidelines. *AORN Journal, 88*(2), 184-196.

Styer, K.S. (2007). Development of a unit-based practice committee: A form of shared governance. *AORN Journal, 86*(1), 85-93.

> **"Go To" Activity — Skill Building**
>
> Participate in an audit for your department. Offer to help analyze the data and report the results to staff.
>
> Volunteer to sit on the quality improvement committee for your facility.
>
> Present a quality improvement or best practice article at your department journal club.

Module 4: Facilitating Professional Behavior

As members of a self-regulated profession, we are accountable to society for our colleagues' practice as well as our own. When disruptive behavior or unsafe practice from any source jeopardizes patient or staff safety, we are obligated to take action.

Competency Outcomes

To successfully complete the activities in this module, you will need to be able to:

1. Choose nursing actions that support patient advocacy.
2. Select behaviors that reflect commitment to professional nursing practice.

Recommended Reading

Alexander's Care of the Patient in Surgery. (2011, 14th ed.), Chapter 30: Workplace issues and staff safety.

Perioperative Standards and Recommended Practices. (2013):
- Exhibit B: Perioperative explications for the ANA code of ethics for nurses, pp. 21-42.
- Standards of perioperative nursing, pp. 3-17.

AORN. (2011). Position Statement: Creating a practice environment of safety. Retrieved March 15, 2013, from http://www.aorn.org/Clinical_Practice/Position_Statements/Position_Statements.aspx.

AORN. (April 2008). Position statement: Criminalization of human errors in the perioperative setting. Retrieved March 15, 2013, from http://www.aorn.org/Clinical_Practice/Position_Statements/Position_Statements.aspx.

Berry and Kohn's Operating Room Technique. (2013, 12th ed.), Section 1: Fundamentals of theory and practice; Chapter 6: Administration of perioperative patient services.

Key Words

Chain of command, collegiality, ethics, healthy work environment, horizontal violence, just culture, lateral violence, patient advocate, professional standards

Activity — Clinical Scenario

R.S., a certified registered nurse anesthetist, has been practicing as an anesthesia care provider for eight years in the same hospital. R.S. has always been very conscientious in his practice (e.g., conducting thorough preoperative patient interviews, setting up his equipment early, collaborating with all members of the surgical team).

During the past six months, you and other staff members have noticed a change in R.S.'s behavior. He frequently comes to work "just-in-time" and has been late on some occasions. He has become increasingly impatient with patients and coworkers and sometimes appears distracted during longer cases. In addition, the postanesthesia care unit (PACU) nurses are reporting that R.S.'s patients require more pain medication than in the past.

Today, you are assigned to a right hemicolectomy, and R.S. is the anesthesia care provider. Midway through the case, you see R.S. has his head down on the anesthesia machine and appears to be asleep.

1. What actions must be taken?

2. What are your professional and ethical obligations?

> **"Go To" Activity — Check It Out!**
>
> Go to Question #13, Healthy work environment, under the Perioperative question of the week tab on your CD for an additional critical-thinking question.

Additional Reading/Resources

AORN. (2007). Human factors toolkit. Retrieved March 15, 2013, from http://www.aorn.org/Secondary.aspx?id=20893. *This resource is for AORN members only.*

Bigony, L., Lipke, T.G., Lundberg, A., McGraw, C.A., et al.(2009). Lateral violence in the perioperative setting. *AORN Journal, 89*(4), 688-700.

Costello, J., Clarke, C., Gravely, G., D'Agostino-Rose, et al. (2011). Working together to build a respectful workplace: Transforming OR culture. *AORN Journal, 93*(1), 115-126.

Hamlin, L. (2009). The OR and a "just culture." *AORN Journal, 90*(4), 495-498.

Kirchner, B. (2009). Safety: Addressing inappropriate behavior in the perioperative workplace. *AORN Journal, 90*(2), 177-180.

Marshall, D.A., & Manus, D.A. (2007). A team training program using human factors to enhance patient safety. *AORN Journal, 88*(6), 994-1011.

McNamara, S. A. (2010). Workplace violence and its effect on patient safety. *AORN Journal, 90*(2), 677-682.

Shumaker, R., & Hickey, P. (2006). Medication diversion in the perioperative setting. *AORN Journal, 83*(3), 745-749.

Chapter Summary

Professionalism in nursing is a personal commitment to patient care based on evidence-based best practices; maintaining currency with changes in the patient population, technology, and the health care environment; and participating actively in the profession through professional organizations. In today's dynamic perioperative environment and diversity of practice settings, the perioperative nurse should continually update and maintain the requisite knowledge and skills as a competent care provider to meet his or her individual professional responsibilities to patients, the profession, and society.

Glossary

Accountability — Being answerable for the consequences/outcomes of one's performance or non-performance of a task, project, or decision for which one is responsible.

Autonomy — In the context of health care, autonomy is the patient's self-determination or ability and power to make his or her own decisions regarding health care.

Beneficence — Doing good; the duty to benefit.

Board of nursing — State governmental agencies that are responsible for the regulation of nursing practice.

Community standard — The practice norm in a specific community, based on resources and the expectations of the consumer.

Competency — The knowledge, skills, and interpersonal abilities needed to fulfill the requirements of the job.

Empirical evidence— Information gathered using the five senses.

Ethical practice —- Nursing practice that encompasses ethical principles, follows the ANA Code of Ethics, and meets society's expectations of ethical behavior.

Ethics — Principles of conduct governing an individual or group.

Evidence-based practice — A problem-solving approach to clinical decision making within a health care organization that integrates the best available scientific evidence with the best available experiential (patient and practitioner) evidence; considers internal and external influences on practice; and encourages critical thinking in the judicious application of such evidence to care of the individual patient, patient population, or system (Newhouse, et al., 2005).

Explication — Explanation.

Information literacy — The ability to access, evaluate, and ethically use information.

Nonmaleficence — In the context of health care, acting in a way as to not harm the patient.

Nurse practice act — Regulations outlined by state boards of nursing that define a nurse's scope of practice.

"Professional culture"/culture of professionalism — An environment that encourages and rewards professional behavior, including academic and continuing education, participation in quality improvement and shared governance, involvement in professional organizations, etc.

Quality improvement — Examining processes with the goal of improving them.

Regulation — Rules adopted by administrative agencies (e.g., state boards of nursing) to administer and regulate the profession.

Responsibility — Ownership of a task, project, or assignment.

Scope of practice — Legal delineation of tasks that a nurse can do dependent upon level of education and licensure as determined by the state board of nursing.

Standard of practice — Delineation of best practices based on research evidence and expert opinion, usually targeting specific patient populations.

Statute — Law enacted by the legislature.

References

American Nurses Association (ANA). (2010). *Nursing Scope and Standards of Practice.* Silver Spring, MD: American Nurses Association.

American Nurses Association (ANA). (2003). *Nursing's Social Policy Statement.* Silver Spring, MD: American Nurses Association.

American Nurses Association (ANA). (2001). *Code of Ethics for Nurses with Interpretive Statements.* Silver Spring, MD: American Nurses Association.

AORN. (2013). Exhibit B: Perioperative explications for the ANA Code of Ethics for nurses. In *Perioperative Standards and Recommended Practices.* Denver: AORN, Inc.

AORN. (2013). Standards of perioperative nursing. In *Perioperative Standards and Recommended Practices.* Denver: AORN, Inc.

Newhouse, R., Dearholt, S., Poe, S., Pugh, L.C., & White, K. (2005). *The Johns Hopkins Nursing Evidence-based Practice Model*. Baltimore, MD: The Johns Hopkins Hospital & Johns Hopkins University School of Nursing.

Phillips, N. (2013). *Berry and Kohn's Operating Room Technique* (12th ed.). St. Louis: Mosby.

Phippen, M.L., Ulmer, B.C., & Wells, M.P. (2009). *Competency for Safe Patient Care During Operative and Invasive Procedures*. Denver: CCI.

Rothrock, J.C. (Ed.). (2007). *Alexander's Care of the Patient in Surgery* (13th ed.). St. Louis: Mosby.

U.S. Department of Justice, Drug Enforcement Administration, Office of Diversion Control. Drug Addiction in Health Care Professionals. Retrieved Feb. 27, 2013, from http://www.deadiversion .usdoj.gov/pubs/brochures/drug_hc.htm.

Answers to Chapter 9 Activities

Module 1: Principles of social policy — Pages 253-255

Activity — Matching

Match the agency with the service it provides:

Association of periOperative Registered Nurses (AORN) - *H*

Centers for Disease Control and Prevention (CDC) - *D*

Centers for Medicare and Medicaid services (CMS) - *B*

Food and Drug Administration (FDA) - *G*

Health Information Portability and Accountability Act (HIPAA) - *C*

The Joint Commission (TJC) - *E*

State board of nursing - *I*

Surgical Care Improvement Project (SCIP) - *F*

Occupational Safety and Health Administration (OSHA) - *A*

Source: Phippen, M. L., Ulmer, B.C., & Wells, M.P. (2009). *Competency for Safe Patient Care During Operative and Invasive Procedures*. Chapter 4. Denver: CCI.

Module 3: Participation in quality improvement activities — Pages 258-259

Activity — Critical thinking

Write the step in the appropriate section for the quality improvement project:

Plan   Do   Study   Act

Do - Data was collected for 3 months by staff in 0730 cases. An audit tool was completed. The top 5 reasons for a late start were analyzed.

Study - Data showed that most cases were late due to insufficient staff to handle volume of patients in pre-admissions testing for day-of laboratory work.

Act - Steps to address findings include:
* Possibility of increasing number of pre-admission staff for morning shift
* Assess workload to determine tasks that could be delegated to another person

Plan - The objective of this project is to decrease the number of late start 0730 cases. Promoting efficient use of time will allow the following cases to also begin on time, increase patient and surgeon satisfaction, and decrease the amount of overtime for staff. Data will be collected related to late starts, type of case, surgeon, and cause of late start.

Source: Phippen, M.L., Ulmer, B.C., & Wells, M.P. (2009). *Competency for Safe Patient Care During Operative and Invasive Procedures*, pp. 47-49. Denver: CCI.

Module 4: Facilitating professional behavior — Pages 260-261

Activity — Clinical Scenario

R.S., a certified registered nurse anesthetist, has been practicing as an anesthesia care provider for eight years in the same hospital. R.S. has always been very conscientious in his practice (e.g., conducting thorough preoperative patient interviews, setting up his equipment early, collaborating with all members of the surgical team).

During the past six months, you and other staff members have noticed a change in R.S.'s behavior. He frequently comes to work "just-in-time" and has been late on some occasions. He has become increasingly impatient with patients and coworkers and sometimes appears distracted during longer cases. In addition, the postanesthesia care unit (PACU) nurses are reporting that R.S.'s patients require more pain medication than in the past.

Today, you are assigned to a right hemicolectomy, and R.S. is the anesthesia care provider. Midway through the case, you see R.S. has his head down on the anesthesia machine and appears to be asleep.

1. What actions must be taken?
Responses may vary but should contain the following key points:

First and foremost, action must be taken to protect the patient. Notify the charge nurse and the supervising anesthesiologist of the situation so that patient care will not be compromised. Second, you also have an obligation to R.S. to report the situation to his supervisor, so R.S. can be evaluated and receive (or refuse) the appropriate intervention.

2. What are your professional and ethical obligations?

The risk of harm to the patient must be removed. You have a professional and ethical obligation to report your observations immediately to the anesthesiologist supervising R.S. You also should report the situation to your manager following your facility chain of command, because the situation has facility-wide ramifications. The anesthesiologist is responsible for taking action to protect the patient by removing R.S. from the case and replacing him with a capable anesthesia care provider. Perioperative nurses should be aware of various programs and resources available to health care providers affected by mental and physical illness or by personal circumstances (e.g., substance abuse, addiction) that impair their ability to perform the duties of the job.

Source: AORN. (2013). Exhibit B: Perioperative explications for the ANA Code of ethics for nurses, pp. 30-31. In *Perioperative Standards and Recommended Practices*. Denver: AORN, Inc.

APPENDICES

Appendix A: CNOR Exam Study Plan

The Competency & Credentialing Institute often receives requests for information on how to study and what to study when preparing for the CNOR exam. The following information is being offered as an example of how to organize topics and references in developing a study plan. Subjects are arranged by their relationship to commonly encountered perioperative tasks, knowledge, and abilities. The key words can be used to further identify not only what is included in each topic but also act as a reference for individual learning needs.

This tool may be modified for individuals as a self-paced learning aid or used in group settings as part of a CNOR exam prep curriculum. This plan is to be used as a guide only and is not meant to serve as an exhaustive review of all available literature. Information on specific specialties is not included in this plan. Additional methods and resources for studying should be explored based on the needs and experience of the applicant.

Required Reference

*   AORN's *Perioperative Standards and Recommended Practices*, 2013 Edition

Highly Recommended References (any of the following)

*   *Alexander's Care of the Patient in Surgery*, Jane Rothrock, Editor, 14th Edition, Elsevier, 2011
*   *Berry and Kohn's Operating Room Technique*, Nancymarie Phillips, Editor, 12th Edition, Elsevier, 2013
*   *Competency for Safe Patient Care During Operative and Invasive Procedures,* Mark Phippen, Brenda Ulmer, Maryann Wells, Editors, CCI, 2009

Additional References

*   *Essentials of Perioperative Nursing*, Spry, C., 5th Edition, 2014
*   *Surgical Technology Principles and Practice,* Fuller, JK., 5th Edition, 2010
*   Pathophysiology Textbook – McCance & Huether and Porth are both very good.
*   Laboratory Manual – Mosby is well regarded, but there are many available.

Key

*   Alexander's – *Alexander's Care of the Patient in Surgery* (2011), 14th edition
*   AORN SRP – *Perioperative Standards and Recommended Practices* (2013);
    Position statements may be accessed at http://www.aorn.org/Clinical_Practice/Position_Statements/Position_Statements.aspx
*   Berry & Kohn's – *Berry and Kohn's Operating Room Technique* (2013), 12th edition
*   Phippen, Ulmer & Wells – *Competency for Safe Patient Care During Operative and Invasive Procedures* (2009)

Subject Area/ Domain	Topic/Key Words	Recommended Readings
1: PREOPERATIVE PATIENT ASSESSMENT and DIAGNOSIS	Advanced directives/DNR Age/culturally specific assessment Anatomy/physiology Nursing diagnosis Pre-op testing: 　Diagnostic studies 　Laboratory results Pain Pathophysiology Pharmacology Universal Protocol Surgical consent	• AORN SRP: Section 1, II; Position statement: DNR • Phippen, Ulmer & Wells: Chapters 2, 5, 6, 12, 18, 36 • Alexander's: Chapters 1, 2, 4, 9, 25, 26, 29; Unit II: Surgical interventions • Berry and Kohn's: Chapters 2, 3, 7-9, 11-13, 21, 23, 25, 30
2: IDENTIFY EXPECTED OUTCOMES and DEVELOP AN INDIVIDUALIZED PLAN OF CARE	Age-specific needs Patient response to surgery (behavioral/physical) Communication/hand offs Community/facility resources Disease processes Legal/ethical responsibilities/ patient rights Nursing process Perioperative safety PNDS Patient/family education needs/ resources Transcultural nursing theory	• AORN SRP: Section I, Exhibit B; II, III • Phippen, Ulmer & Wells: Chapters 1, 2, 5, 18 • Alexander's: Chapters 1, Unit II; Unit III • Berry and Kohn's: Chapters 2, 7, 9, 11, 21
3: INTRAOPERATIVE ACTIVITIES	Anatomy/physiology Anesthesia agents/management Aseptic technique Documentation Environmental cleaning Environmental management Ergonomics Expected outcomes Hazardous materials Implants/explants Intraoperative blood salvage Instruments, supplies/equipment/manufacturers' recommendations Medication administration Pain management Patient advocacy Pharmacology Physiologic response to surgery Potential complications Prevention of retained surgical items/counts	• AORN SRP: Units II and III; Position statements: Noise in the perioperative practice setting; Creating a practice environment of safety • Phippen, Ulmer & Wells: Chapters 4-17, Section III, Section IV • Alexander's: Chapters 2-8, 30; Unit II, Unit III • Berry and Kohn's: Chapters 2, 7, 10-13, 15, 16, 19-29, 31; Section 12

Subject Area/ Domain	Topic/Key Words	Recommended Readings
3: INTRAOPERATIVE ACTIVITIES *(continued)*	Principles of infection control/ standard and transmission-based Principles of patient/personnel safety Principles of wound healing/ skin integrity/wound classifications Problem solving/critical thinking skills Professional standards of care Regulatory guidelines Skin antisepsis Specimens Surgical procedures Universal Protocol	
4: COMMUNICATION	Collaborative reporting/critical values Communication techniques Confidentiality Interdisciplinary plan of care Interviewing techniques Medication reconciliation Universal Protocol	• AORN SRP: Transfer of patient care information; Perioperative health care information; Medication safety • Phippen, Ulmer & Wells: Chapter 4 • Alexander's: Chapters 1, 2 • Berry and Kohn's: Chapters 2, 3, 6, 7, 21
5: TRANSFER of CARE	Coordination between interdisciplinary care services Documentation Patient education Post-op complications Post-op follow-up Transfer of care criteria	• AORN SRP: Transfer of patient care information • Phippen, Ulmer & Wells: Chapters 6, 18, 37, 38 • Alexander's: Chapters 2, 9, 25, 26; Unit II • Berry and Kohn's: Chapters 11, 25, 30
6: CLEANING, DISINFECTING, PACKAGING, STERILIZING, TRANSPORTING and STORING INSTRUMENTS/ SUPPLIES	Documentation Environmental conditions for sterilization/storage Handling/disposition of hazardous/biohazardous materials Infection prevention/standard/ transmission-based Microbiology Principles of cleaning/disinfection Principles of packaging/sterilization Principles of transporting/storage Professional/regulatory standards	• AORN SRP: High level disinfection; Prevention of transmissible infections; Cleaning/processing flexible endoscopes; Cleaning/care of instruments/powered equipment; Sterilization; Selection/use of packaging systems; Safe environment of care; Guidance statement: Role of the health care industry representative • Phippen, Ulmer & Wells: Chapters 9, 11, 14 • Alexander's: Chapters 3, 7, 30 • Berry and Kohn's: Chapters 13-18

Subject Area/ Domain	Topic/Key Words	Recommended Readings
7: EMERGENCY SITUATIONS	Anaphylaxis Cardiac arrest Fire Malignant hyperthermia Natural disasters Terrorism Trauma	• AORN SRP: Safe environment of care; Managing patient receiving moderate sedation; Prevention of transmissible infections; pp. 129, 149-151, 220-224 • Phippen, Ulmer & Wells: pp. 96, 126-127, 158-164, 408-415, 424-428, 626-627; Chapter 32 • Alexander's: pp. 32-33, 40-42, 64-66, 98, 104, 128, 140-141, 235-237, 272-277, 278-280, 369, 673, 1278-1280, Chapters 23-25, 27 • Berry and Kohn's: pp. 20-21, 85, 126, 224-226, 230-231, 248, 251, 513, 575-576, 682-683, 733, 744, 765, 800-801, 815-816, 919-920; Chapter 31
8: MANAGEMENT OF PERSONNEL, SERVICES, and MATERIALS	Acquiring equipment, supplies, and personnel Basic management/delegation Environmental consciousness Product evaluation/cost containment Role of health care industry representative Scope of practice Visitors/students	• AORN SRP: Section 1, Exhibit B; Sterilization; Guidance statements: Perioperative staffing; Safe on-call practices; Role of health care industry representative AORN Position statements: Responsibility for mentoring; Environmental responsibility; Allied health care providers; Value of clinical learning activities • Phippen, Ulmer & Wells: Chapter 4 • Alexander's: Chapters 1, 2 • Berry and Kohn's: pp. 213, 300-301, 325-326; Chapters 1-4, 6
9: PROFESSIONAL ACCOUNTABILITY	Competence standards Evidence-based practice Disruptive behavior Performance improvement Regulatory standards Research Resources for professional growth Scope of practice	• AORN SRP: Section I, Exhibit B; Position statements: Criminalization of human errors; Creating a practice environment of safety • Phippen, Ulmer & Wells: Chapters 1, 3, 4 • Alexander's: Chapters 1, 30 • Berry and Kohn's: Section 1; Chapters 4, 6

My Personal Study Plan

With the information you found in this *Guide*, use this and the following page to start your own personal study plan. Include timelines, learning needs, additional references and resources, frequently used web sites — anything you need to help organize your schedule and maximize your study time.

My Personal Study Plan, *continued*

Appendix B: Domains for the CNOR Exam

Domain 1: Preoperative Patient Assessment and Diagnosis

Questions on the exam will deal with the following topics:
1. Advance directives and do-not-resuscitate (DNR)
2. Age and culturally appropriate health assessment techniques
3. Anatomy and physiology
4. Approved nursing diagnoses (North American Nursing Diagnosis Association [NANDA], *Perioperative Nursing Data Set* [PNDS])
5. Cultural/diversity assessment
6. Diagnostic procedures and results
7. Pain measurement techniques
8. Pathophysiology
9. Pharmacology
10. Universal Protocol
11. Surgical consent

Required Elements of Domain 1
- Confirm patient identity with two patient identifiers, procedure and operative site, side/site marking
- Verify the surgical consent
- Conduct an individualized physical assessment including but not limited to skin integrity and mobility deficits
- Use age and culturally appropriate health assessment and interview techniques
- Collect, analyze, and prioritize patient data (allergies, lab values, other medical conditions, previous relevant surgical history, chart review, NPO status)
- Review medication history (preoperative medications, home medications, alternative and herbal supplements, medical marijuana use, alcohol use, recreational drug use)
- Perform a pain assessment
- Confirm advance directive and DNR status
- Formulate nursing diagnoses
- Document preoperative assessment

Domain 2: Identify Expected Outcomes and Develop an Individualized Plan of Care

Questions on the exam will deal with the following topics:
1. Age-specific needs
2. Behavioral responses to the operative/invasive experience
3. Communication skills
4. Community and institutional resources
5. Disease processes
6. Legal and ethical responsibilities and implications for patient care
7. Nursing process
8. Patient rights and responsibilities
9. Perioperative safety
10. *Perioperative Nursing Data Set* (PNDS)
11. Physiologic responses to the surgical experience
12. Resources for patient/family education
13. Transcultural nursing theory, including cultural and ethnic influences, family patterns, spirituality, and other related practices
14. Teaching/learning needs of patients and families

Required Elements of Domain 2
- Identify potential physiologic responses (e.g., infection, tissue perfusion, thermal regulation) to the operative/invasive experience
- Assess behavioral responses of patient and family (comfort, anxiety, medication, pain management, cultural and spiritual issues) to the operative/invasive procedure
- Incorporate age-specific needs into the plan of care
- Specify diversity needs and requirements (language barriers, attire)
- Perform preoperative teaching
- Collaborate with the interdisciplinary health care team
- Appraise legal and ethical guidelines related to patient care
- Apply principles of perioperative safety (e.g., chemical exposure, radiation, fire, laser, positioning to plan of care)
- Identify and communicate measurable patient outcomes across the continuum of care (hand-offs)

Domain 3: Intraoperative Activities

Questions on the exam will deal with the following topics:

1. Anatomy and physiology
2. Anesthesia management and anesthetic agents
3. Aseptic technique
4. Documentation of all nursing interventions
5. Environmental cleaning (spills, room turnover, terminal cleaning)
6. Environmental factors (temperature, humidity, air exchange, noise, traffic patterns)
7. Ergonomics and body mechanics
8. Equipment use per manufacturers' instructions
9. Expected outcomes related to identified interventions
10. Implants and explants (handling, tracking, sterilization)
11. Intraoperative blood salvage
12. Instruments, supplies, and equipment relating to surgical procedure
13. Medication management, including the seven rights
14. Pain management
15. Patients' rights
16. Pharmacology
17. Physiologic responses to the surgical experience
18. Potential complications
19. Preoperative patient preparation activities
20. Prevention of retained surgical items (counts)
21. Principles of infection control
22. Principles of patient/personnel safety
23. Principles of wound healing
24. Problem solving skills
25. Professional standards of care
26. Regulatory guidelines
27. Requirements for handling hazardous materials
28. Requirements for handling specimens
29. Role as a patient advocate
30. Skin antisepsis
31. Smoke plumes
32. Standard and transmission-based precautions
33. Surgical procedure
34. Universal Protocol
35. Wound classification

Required Elements of Domain 3

- Perform Universal Protocol
- Assist with anesthesia management
- Monitor and evaluate the effects of pharmacologic and anesthetic agents
- Label solutions, medications, and medication containers

- Perform proper patient positioning
- Utilize proper body mechanics
- Prepare the surgical site
- Maintain the dignity, modesty, and privacy of the patient
- Select procedure-specific protective barrier materials
- Assess expiration date and package integrity of products
- Maintain a sterile field utilizing aseptic technique
- Perform counts
- Optimize physiologic responses of the patient to the operative/invasive procedure
- Conduct and document intraoperative blood salvage
- Optimize behavioral responses of patient and family (e.g., comfort, anxiety, operative procedure, medication, pain management, cultural, spiritual and ethical issues) to operative/invasive procedure
- Monitor and maintain patient and personnel safety (chemical, fire, smoke plumes, radiation, laser, positioning)
- Identify and control environmental factors (noise, temperature, traffic)
- Test and use equipment according to manufacturers' recommendations
- Confirm, prepare, and present implants to sterile field
- Prepare explants for final disposition
- Prepare, label, and transport specimens
- Perform or supervise environmental cleaning for room turnover, spills, and terminal cleaning
- Utilize professional standards of care
- Utilize problem-solving skills to facilitate patient care
- Protect patient confidentiality
- Advocate for and protect patients' rights
- Maintain accurate patient records/documentation related to plan of care and nursing interventions

Domain 4: Communication

Questions on the exam will deal with the following topics:
1. Collaborative reporting to interdisciplinary health care providers (e.g., critical lab values, medical condition, medications, allergies, implants/implantable devices, hand-off, read back verbal orders, communication barriers)
2. Communication techniques
3. Interdisciplinary plan of care
4. Interviewing techniques
5. Medication reconciliation
6. Proper use of documentation tools
7. Regulatory guidelines (e.g., confidentiality)
8. Universal Protocol

Required Elements of Domain 4
- Identify patient barriers to communication and incorporate effective solutions
- Communicate patient status and changes to the interdisciplinary health care providers (critical lab values, medical condition, medications, allergies, implants/implantable devices)
- Utilize hand-offs and read back for verbal orders
- Maintain patient confidentiality
- Provide information to the patient/family according to HIPAA guidelines (status, updates)

Domain 5: Transfer of Care

Questions on the exam will deal with the following topics:
1. Coordination of interdisciplinary care services
2. Documentation of the transfer of care
3. Patient postoperative follow-up communication following regulatory guidelines
4. Perioperative patient education techniques
5. Postoperative complications
6. Transfer of care criteria

Required Elements of Domain 5
- Evaluate patient status to facilitate transfer to the next level of care (PACU, ICU, home)
- Collaborate with interdisciplinary services (nutrition, wound care, social work, visiting nurse, referrals, transportation)
- Document perioperative education
- Document transfer of care
- Provide and document post discharge follow-up communication according to regulatory guidelines

Domain 6: Cleaning, Disinfecting, Packaging, Sterilizing, Transporting, and Storing Instruments and Supplies

Questions on the exam will deal with the following topics:

1. Documentation requirements for sterilization, biological and chemical monitoring
2. Environmental conditions of sterilization and storage areas
3. Handling and disposition of biohazardous materials (e.g., blood, infectious pathogens such as Creutzfeldt-Jakob Disease [CJD])
4. Handling and disposition of hazardous materials (e.g., chemotherapy drugs, radioactive materials)
5. Microbiology and infection prevention
6. Regulatory requirements for tracking of materials and instruments brought in from outside the facility
7. Principles of cleaning and disinfection
8. Principles of packaging and sterilizing
9. Principles of transporting and storage
10. Professional and regulatory standards (AORN Standards and Recommended Practices, Occupational Safety and Health Administration [OSHA], Centers for Disease Control and Prevention [CDC], Association for the Advancement of Medical Instrumentation [AAMI])
11. Standard and transmission-based precautions

Required Elements of Domain 6

- Use appropriate personal protective equipment (PPE)
- Choose the appropriate method for cleaning and disinfection of contaminated equipment and instruments
- Select appropriate packaging
- Determine appropriate sterilization method
- Select appropriate method(s) for biological/chemical monitoring
- Select appropriate methods for transporting and storing processed supplies and instruments
- Monitor environmental conditions (e.g., humidity, temperature) of sterilization and storage areas
- Document actions related to cleaning, disinfecting, packaging, sterilizing, transporting, and storing instruments and supplies
- Describe appropriate handling and disposition of hazardous materials (e.g., chemotherapy drugs, radioactive materials)
- Describe appropriate handling and disposition of biohazardous materials (e.g., blood, infectious pathogens such as Creutzfeldt-Jakob Disease [CJD])
- Manage materials and instruments brought in from outside the facility

Domain 7: Emergency Situations

Questions on the exam will deal with the following topics:

1. Identification of, preparation for, and nursing interventions related to:
   a. Anaphylaxis
   b. Cardiac arrest
   c. Environmental hazards (e.g., fire)
   d. Malignant hyperthermia (MH)
   e. Natural disasters (e.g., hurricanes, floods, tornados)
   f. Terrorism
   g. Trauma
2. Roles of interdisciplinary health care team members

Required Elements of Domain 7

- Function as a member of the interdisciplinary health care team in the prevention or management of:
  - Anaphylaxis
  - Cardiac arrest
  - Environmental hazards (e.g., fire)
  - Malignant hyperthermia (MH)
  - Natural disasters (e.g., hurricanes, floods, tornados)
  - Terrorism
  - Trauma

Domain 8: Management of Personnel, Services, and Materials

Questions on the exam will deal with the following topics:
1. Acquiring equipment, supplies, and personnel for proper room preparation
2. Basic management techniques and delegation
3. Environmental consciousness (go green)
4. Principles of product evaluation and cost containment
5. Role of the health care industry representative (HCIR)
6. Role of non-OR personnel (e.g., visitors, students) in the OR
7. Scope of practice

Required Elements of Domain 8
*   Utilize critical thinking skills to anticipate the needs for and acquire equipment, supplies, and personnel
*   Delegate perioperative tasks to appropriate personnel according to regulatory agencies' standards
*   Monitor and implement cost-containment measures
*   Practice environmental consciousness (go green)
*   Supervise, educate, and mentor health care team members
*   Manage health care industry representative (HCIR) presence in the OR
*   Supervise non-OR personnel, including visitors and students
*   Participate in product evaluation/selection

Domain 9: Professional Accountability

Questions on the exam will deal with the following topics:

1. Regulatory standards and voluntary guidelines (AORN Standards and Recommended Practices, OSHA, ANA Code of Ethics for Nurses with Explications for Perioperative Nurses, state nurse practice act)
2. Scope of practice
3. Resources for professional growth
4. Competence standards in perioperative nursing practice
5. Quality improvement activities for research
6. Quality improvement activities for evidence based practice
7. Quality improvement activities for performance improvement
8. Responsibilities regarding impaired and/or disruptive behavior (patient/family, interdisciplinary health care team members)

Required Elements of Domain 9

- Function within scope of practice
- Demonstrate competence in perioperative nursing practice
- Uphold and act upon ethical and professional standards
- Assess personal limitations and seek assistance as needed
- Identify and utilize resources for professional growth (e.g., shared governance activities, hospital committees, professional organizations)
- Identify quality improvement activities that promote performance improvement, evidence based practice, and research
- Choose appropriate actions when intervening with impaired/disruptive behavior in patients and/or family members, health care team members

Appendix C: CCI CNOR 2013 Test Specifications

Domains	2013 Final % of items per domain	2013 Final # of items per domain
1. Preoperative Patient Assessment and Diagnosis	14%	26
2. Identify Expected Outcomes and Develop an Individualized Plan of Care	9%	17
3. Intraoperative Activities	31%	57
4. Communication	9%	17
5. Transfer of Care	5%	9
6. Cleaning, Disinfecting, Packaging, Sterilizing, Transporting, and Storing Instruments and Supplies	12%	22
7. Emergency Situations	8%	15
8. Management of Personnel, Services, and Materials	6%	11
9. Professional Accountability	6%	11
TOTAL	*100%*	*185*

Appendix D: Regulatory and Health Care Agencies, Professional Organizations

All website addresses were current as of April 10, 2013.

American Nurses Association (ANA)
http://nursingworld.org/

Association for the Advancement of Medical Instrumentation (AAMI)
http://www.aami.org/

Association of periOperative Registered Nurses (AORN)
http://www.aorn.org

Centers for Disease Control and Prevention (CDC)
http://www.cdc.gov/

Centers for Medicare and Medicaid Services
http://www.cms.gov/

Healthcare Infection Control Practices Advisory Committee (HICPAC)
http://www.cdc.gov/hicpac/index.html

Institute for Healthcare Improvement (IHI)
http://www.ihi.org/

Institutes of Medicine. (Nov., 1999). To err is human: Building a safer health system.
http://www.iom.edu/~/media/Files/Report%20Files/1999/To-Err-is-Human/
To%20Err%20is%20Human%201999%20%20report%20brief.pdf

The Joint Commission
http://www.jointcommission.org/

National Institute for Occupational Safety and Health (NIOSH)
http://www.cdc.gov/niosh/

Surgical Care Improvement Project (SCIP)
http://www.ihi.org/explore/SSI/Pages/default.aspx

U.S. Department of Labor, Occupational Safety and Health Administration (OSHA).
http://www.osha.gov/

NOTES

NOTES

NOTES

NOTES